CANDIDA

AND RESTORE YOUR
IMMUNE SYSTEM

CONQUER
CANDIDA

AND RESTORE YOUR
IMMUNE SYSTEM

— by —

Jack Tips
N.D., Ph.D.

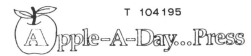
Apple-A-Day...Press

Cover design by Charles Harvey
Cover drawing of flame person by Kathy Brown.

Printed in the United States
Eighteenth Printing, 2002

Published by

Apple-A-Day...Press

1500 Village West #77
Austin, Texas 78733-1977
512-328-3996
512-263-7787 fax
apple-a-day@austin.rr.com

www.apple-a-daypress.com

Contact the Author:
www.jacktips.com

*This information is presented in good will
for informational and educational purposes.*

ISBN 0-929167-00-7

When we realize that through ignorance
of Natural Law
We create our illness,
It must be more than acknowledging
Our self-responsibility;
We must know
That we can just as assuredly
Create our wellness.

Jack Tips, 1985

CONTENTS

From the Publisher . . .

PREFACE TO THE
1989 EDITION

It's been four years since the initial research "Conquer Candida" was published. We estimate that more than 5000 people have been helped by their understanding and application of the information provided by this research.

To decide whether or not to update and reprint this information, we perused the bookstores to see what breakthroughs had occurred in the last four years, and see if this particular research was outdated by the mass market books so readily available.

Frankly, we were disturbed by what we found. Although there were new books about controlling candida on the market as well as the basic primers (*The Yeast Connection, The Yeast Syndrome*) which seem to be on everyone's reference shelves, there was no new information! All we found was the same information that has been out for quite sometime now — information that only speaks of possibly controlling candida and nothing so bold as to speak of conquering it!

Evidentally candida is still an important topic (people's lives depend on their immune integrity!) but no-one has anything new to say about it, or the publishers of such books don't think the public can handle a stronger dose of the true story.

Conquer Candida and Restore Your Immune System still provides the most current, most innovative, most insightful, most provocative information available.

Needless to say, we feel obligated to reprint this material and are proud to offer this milestone in naturopathic philosophy and guide to better health.

You'll find information and tools to truly improve your health as well as understand how to build a future for yourself and your family whether you have candida or not.

Apple-A-Day Press is dedicated to providing information on natural healing and wellness based on clinical experience — the proving ground for what really works — and keen insights into the frontiers of wholistic health.

We expect you'll be intrigued, entertained, outraged and excited by our offerings, and find the tools to build a vibrant, natural health. That's what we expect in our materials and what you can expect from Apple-A-Day Press!

CONQUER CANDIDA
AND RESTORE YOUR IMMUNE SYSTEM

INTRODUCTION

From a philosophical perspective, infection with the "disease" Candidiasis* may be the most profound BLESSING for mankind in the 20th Century! It may be difficult to understand how a disease can be a blessing, particularly when you see people with the many symptoms of pathogenic* Candida albicans* (fatigue, allergies, premenstrual syndrome, depression, intestinal bloating, chronic vaginal infections), but this condition puts several aspects of our life-style under close scrutiny and demands a radical departure from our current course. And if our success in understanding and conquering candida as an illness becomes a model by which to live a joyous, healthful, fulfilled life; then it is indeed a profound blessing.

From a less lofty perspective — one that admits humankind will probably not make the necessary changes in diet, attitude, health care, and life-style — then it might be too late already. Candidiasis will remain the silent specter, snapping at the immune system's heels, driving the body to ruin.

Ultimately the decision belongs to the individual. If you have a pioneering spirit and a strong survival instinct, you will consider this material open-mindedly, and you too can conquer candida. But understand right now that to conquer candida requires a total health approach. This means restoration of the immune system, endocrine system, and digestive/eliminative/hepatic (liver) system.

Here is a quick definition for those unfamiliar with exactly what candida is. Candida is a microbe known as yeast, which is a normal inhabitant of the body. For a variety of reasons (discussed in this material), it can become a pathogen — a disease-causing fungus that feeds on the body and weakens the immune system leaving a person susceptible to allergies, AIDS, chronic fatigue (Epstein-Barr), herpes, and many other illnesses.

Words denoted with an asterix (*) are defined in the glossary.

1

Candida is called a disease because the fungal aspect is an infection. Actually candidiasis is only a SYMPTOM of a weakened immune system. The real problem is weak or overburdened immunity, not the "bug" candida.

So far, treatments for candidiasis have not been very effective. The best ones are only controlling it, doing little to repair the damage already done. This is like treading water in hungry shark territory. The person's not drowning, but danger is imminent. This material will present NEW tools for conquering candida and a three-step plan for getting out of the water. It will also point out the pathway for staying out of troubled waters once therapies are discontinued.

In this dissertation, our eye of scrutiny will examine a cornerstone of today's medical practice — antibiotics and hormonal/chemical drugs. It will also look at breast-feeding, diet, stress, and various nutritional alternatives. Our focus on candida will allow us to expand our awareness of basic health processes to a greater degree of truth. To conquer candida, we must address some basic tenets of nutrition and the laws of Nature that naturopathy* has taught for centuries—the simple laws of working with the body the way the body was designed to work.

It must be said most emphatically that candidiasis can be conquered. This is a powerful statement because most people are fortunate to be able to barely control candida, much less conquer it. There is indeed an answer, but it may not be as simple or convenient as people with unnatural lifestyles wish. There is evidence that once people contract candidiasis, they always have a predisposition towards it. This means that, once conquered, candida can return and is likely to do so if the proper environment is once again provided. We'll take a look at "proper environment," and most importantly, how to avoid it.

Candidiasis is only a symptom that we have gone astray from the natural health processes of the body. And the damage, if caught early, can be corrected. It's true that our medical leaders have led us astray, but ignorance never has been an excuse, and ultimately we must be responsible for our own health and make necessary changes ourselves. Fortunately great strides have been made in nutritional therapies and biological medicine* that provide answers to help people return to a healthy, vibrant life-style.

2

There's one detrimental attitude that must be addressed up front. It's the doom and gloom attitude that some doctors and nutritionists are putting on people with candidiasis. Such attitudes don't help and only get in the way. Let's drop the idea of suffering with restricted diets and crawling through life with reduced energy levels. This doesn't have to be! Let go of the idea that candidiasis is a disease that is beyond control. Such limiting concepts are false.

Also, since the toxic by-products of candida can cause depression and a lack of self confidence, a person's self-defeating attitude can have a bio-chemical basis. This is particularly true of people affected with the Epstein Barr virus (Chronic Fatigue Syndrome). A secondary effect is depression and a belief that there is no help and life is hardly worth living. This is quickly reinforced by doctors who tell these people there is no cure and they must learn to live with chronic fatigue and profound self pity. [Clinically we have found this not to be true because nutritional, herbal, and homeopathic therapies have restored many chronic fatique sufferers in two to three months as evidenced by their return to the workplace, sustained energy, and positive attitudes.

Let's take a new look at candida from beginning to end and we'll learn some things about this "new enemy." We'll discover it's only a symptom of a different problem — and, most importantly, how we can conquer it. The solution is so basic it takes special insight to wade through all the hoopla and find it. But that's what this material is about.

One more point: Candida overgrowth is not really new. Hippocrates (the father of medicine) mentioned it a while back in Greece's golden age. Flare ups called "thrush" and "vaginitis" have been around for centuries — not a common ailment until recently, but one mentioned in some of the older medical, eclectic, and herbology books. But in the past these were considered acute conditions. Candidiasis as we now know it has become a chronic degenerative disease, lingering, smoldering, and slowly destroying the body's vital functions. And TODAY'S VARIETIES OF CANDIDA-TYPE INFECTIONS MAY WELL BE GENETICALLY DIFFERENT THAN PREVIOUSLY KNOWN — MORE VIRULENT AND MORE RESISTANT TO TREATMENT.

3

It is a mistake to consider candidiasis a simple yeast infection. It's not. It is a fungus that may have originated as yeast, but has become a fungus and learned how to attack cells. As a fungus it does not behave like yeast or yeast infection. At this time not much is known about candida and the other members of the albicans family. But such knowledge is not nearly so valuable as an understanding of WHY candida has become such a problem to millions of people. By knowing why, a person is empowered to change, grow, and heal.

CANDIDIASIS: HOW SERIOUS IS THIS DISEASE?

Until recently candidiasis has not been treated very seriously. It was considered a secondary problem because it would flare up when some other ailment taxed the immune system. And once the other ailment was corrected, the candidiasis would also subside. So candida was seldom a primary focus.

As recent as 1987, the medical establishment is officially pooh-poohing candida as an imaginary illness and, of course, failing to acknowledge their responsibility in causing it. This stance continues on into 1989, but more and more doctors are admitting candida is a serious, iatrogenic* disease, particularly in the light of insurmountable evidence. But now, however, it has become a primary concern to millions of people because of its devastating effects on the immune system and a person's ability to continue living.

Yes, candidiasis can be fatal, and often is. The death certificate may say something else, such as "kidney failure," "liver disease," "alzheimer's", "cardiac arrest," "pneumonia," and so forth, but the cell-invasive fungus candida paved the way.

Let's keep our perspective on this point. It is already obvious to many of our nation's leading physicians that candidiasis is real, running out of control, and a major concern and challenge for the whole field of medicine as we know it today. Because the symptoms are so varied, the treatments often ineffective, and the disease itself so elusive, it is quite likely that "candida" is the new buzzword for whatever ails a person [similar to the popularity of hypoglycemia (low blood sugar) in the past decade, with many people assuming they have it just to be in vogue, when they may actually have other difficulties.

Candida certainly is a "jump on the bandwagon" disease, but some doctors estimate that as many as 80% of the population may have yeast/fungus involvement to some degree. It is certainly a major consideration and should not be laughed at as many doctors do in response to the public being more informed than they are. In the late 1960s, it was popular for people to have hypoglycemia (or think they did). Then in the 70s everyone got food allergies. Now

5

in the 80's it's candida. Some wonder if it was candida all along. Others blame our society's life-style and dietary pattern. Others think it's all silly. But by reading this material you'll be able to judge for yourself if you are a candidate for candida involvement, as well as understand the role it plays with hypoglycemia and allergies.

Candidiasis is a prerequisite to AIDS (Acquired Immune Deficiency Syndrome), as it provides the immune weaknesses and distortions of the immune processes. Also, the symbiotic* and competitive parasite Giardia has been found to be a haven for the AIDS virus. According to Dr. Warren Levin, by eliminating both candida and the giardia, the HTLV3 virus loses its habitat and progress can be made to rebuild the level of health.

Keeping in mind that many more people contact AIDS than contract it, this issue is really one of the body's acceptance of it.

What makes one person's body accept AIDS and succumb to the virus, and another person's body successfully reject it? A simple answer is one person has a weak immune system (an environment conducive to accepting pathogenic organisms), and the other person has a strong immune system.

Without too big a leap in logic, we could say that anything that weakens the immune system compromises health and makes a person susceptible to illness including AIDS. Candida weakens the immune system very effectively. So do a host of of other things, but beyond what "ordinary" pathogens do, candida alters and distorts the immune response.

The chain of events runs like this:

STEP ONE: Something challenges the immune system and contributes to the body's immune burden.

STEP TWO: Candida-yeast growth increases, fungal forms (when allowed) further challenge the immune system.

STEP THREE: If the immune system does not meet the entire challenge, fungal forms continue to challenge the immune system, and begin to attack and weaken the immune system.

6

STEP FOUR: Weakened immunity leaves the body prey to other pathogenic organisms, and further candida involvement.

This "normal" sequence of events is not really supposed to occur because the body has very effective systems built in to prevent such degeneration. So what's happened? What are we doing that allows that sequence to occur?

So the real issue of Candidasis, and AIDS for that matter, and all chronic-degenerative diseases is one of personal immune integrity.

The basic question now is this: Is your immune system strong enough to meet the challenges of today's environment, or is it weakened and overtaxed by your personal environment (diet, attitude, smoking, medications, recreational drugs, alcohol, chemical exposure, pollutants, dental fillings, excessive stress, etc.) and thus unable to effectively perform its job?

The following article is a reprint of typical material that tries to refute the validity of Candidiasis as a disease. It is from the May, 1987, "University of California, Berkeley, Wellness Letter" (a pseudo-nutritional mouthpiece for the established medical society.)

Yeast: the root of all evil?

If you read magazines, you may have seen a lot about candidiasis, or "chronic candidiasis hypersensitivity syndrome." What you won't read is that there's no scientific support for this "syndrome." Many species of Candida—most commonly *Candida albicans*, a ubiquitous yeast—live in animals and humans, especially in the mouth, throat, intestine, and vagina. As a rule, they trouble no one, but at times they do cause infection. Many women have experienced a vaginal Candida infection that can be hard to cure, and widespead candidiasis can occur in people who are already extremely ill or on long-term antibiotics.

But Dr. William Crook, author of the bestselling book *The Yeast Connection*, claims that this common yeast is at the root of scores of health problems. He believes that an overgrowth of Candida in a large percentage of the population has led to a marked increase in allergy or sensitivity to Candida and to suppression of the immune system. He blames this overgrowth on the use of antibiotics or birth control pills, exposure to environmental toxins, and especially a diet high in sugar. This suppression of the immune system, he claims, predisposes people to a host of other sensitivities to various foods and chemicals as well as infection. He states that the resulting disorders include depression, hyperactivity, upset stomach, premenstrual syndrome, and even rheumatoid arthritis, cancer, multiple sclerosis, and AIDS.

7

The diagnosis is made by excluding other possible causes of your symptoms. If you've got it, you'll know because you'll respond to the treatment, says Dr. Crook. Treatment can consist of many things, but will probably include elimination of all sugar and yeast—especially bread—from your diet, avoidance of all processed (even frozen) foods, installation of air filters to create "safe" rooms, and giving up cosmetics or any products that contain petrochemcials. You may also be told to take certain antifungal drugs or be given "immunotherapy."

The trouble is that there is no scientific or experimental evidence that any of this theory is valid. True Candida sensitivity is rare and can be diagnosed by a competent allergist. Although many people claim that Dr. Crook's regimen has helped them, this is most likely a "placebo effect"—that is, people are sometimes helped merely by entering a therapeutic relationship. The dangers of following Dr. Crook's advice include the misdiagnosis of what might have been a treatable or curable disease, or the adoption of a diet that might ultimately be unhealthy. Like any theory that claims to solve everything, this one can waste time, energy, and hope. Moreover, antifungal drugs can have life-threatening side effects. "This book can change your life," its author promises. But probably not for the better.

It would be encouraging to report that now in 1989 such ignorance would have been replaced with admission of the widespread effects of Candidiasis and advice on how to avoid it, but the ramifications are evidently too great since they would include an admission that Medicine's allopathic (chemical drug) approach is the CAUSE of Candidiasis and therefore a contributor to the demise of the human immune system.

Most doctors continue to deny Candidiasis, or at best look the other way hoping it will go away. But it is reassuring to know that there are now many doctors who are now recognizing the validity of candida-involvement in their patients and encouraging them to avoid antibiotics and birth control pills; to treat the candida, and to follow more nutritional diets.

Candidiasis is introducing into the medical community the facts that overuse of drugs (antibiotics, steroids) are detrimental and that natural diets can be an important part of a health-recovery program.

Perhaps another BLESSING of Candidiasis might be a curving away of drug-medicine from its destructive course of assuming

8

every ailment of the body is a drug deficiency which can be corrected by a dose of drugs, and a reintroduction of the validity of diet as an essential for health and a way to treat and correct disease. We'll see.

Generally speaking, Candidiasis is a serious concern because it compromises the immune system. We'll discuss this later. Specifically for people whose candida involvement causes their health to be impaired, it is an infection that causes a variety of aggravating symptoms.

SYMPTOMS OF CANDIDIASIS-INVOLVEMENT

Candidiasis can cause life-altering diseases and conditions such as:

acne
allergies
anemia
asthma
catatonic schizophrenia
chemical sensitivities
constipation (chronic)
cold hands and feet
cough
cramps
cystitis
dementia
depression
diabetes
diarrhea (chronic)
drug use tendencies
drunk feeling
earaches
eczema
endometriosis
environmental sensitivities
food sensitivities
gas
headaches
hives

hyperactivity
hypothyroidism
impaired sensory perceptions
(hearing, sight, taste, smell)
irrational fears
joint pain that travels
kidney/bladder infections
lethargy
loss of libido (sex drive)
low self-esteem
menstrual irregularity
memory lapse
migraine headaches
miscarriages
muscle cramps
numbness
obesity
premenstrual syndrome
vaginitis
auto-immune diseases such as
Crohn's
hemolytic anemia
lupus
multiple sclerosis
myasthenia gravis

procrastination	scleroderma
psoriasis	sore throat
rheumatoid arthritis	thrombocytopenic purpura
sarcoidosis	weight gain

Candidiasis is being found to be the disease behind the other diseases. Your understanding of the processes involved in candida proliferation will be your passport to a more secure future for yourself, your family, and perhaps many others.

Before we go into greater detail about the the many symptoms of Candidiasis and how it affects many of the body's systems, let's first become fully acquainted with yeast/fungus so we can understand the big picture before the specifics.

CANDIDA'S (YEAST'S) ROLE IN THE ORDER OF THINGS

Candida albicans starts out as a microorganism known as yeast. Actually it is more accurately defined as a "yeast-like" microorganism. Yeasts are single-cell plants that inundate this planet, meaning they're everywhere. But unlike plants, yeasts do not synthesize sunlight and contain no chlorophyll. They ferment sugars and carbohydrates for their life processes instead. Until recently, yeast caused little need for concern. Occasionally a condition called "thrush" would occur if yeast became too prolific in the oral area.

Actually a better name for candida would be "Albicans" - the name of the whole family of yeasts. "Candida" is the first name, "Albicans" is the family or surname. There are many different kinds of albicans, all of which are quite detrimental to the body when they get out of control. They go by names such as monilia albicans, oidium albicans, and saccaromyces albicans.

So a person's "candidiasis" problem might not be candida but a brother or sister of candida. Common usage has established the wrong name for what's actually bothering some people. And many people are being bothered by more than one member of the albicans family. But common useage prevails and we'll call it all "candida."

Such distinctions may not mean much to the average person, but it's quite significant to the microbiologist keeping track of what genetic material is changing into what pathogenic disease. And with medical science getting very specific with their chemicals, a drug that kills Monilia albicans may be completely ineffective against Candida albicans, and may even cause it to proliferate. This is one reason why some people have a disease very similiar to candidiasis, but may not respond very well to medical treatment. (On the other hand, less-specific herbal treatment covers a wider variety of fungi and thus presents a viable alternative to whatever the problem may actually be.) This is one reason why the natural therapies have been so successful in helping people.

Candida is a shape-changer. It's genetic code (DNA — deoxyribonucleic acid) changes within itself, giving it completely different characteristics. Scientists use descriptive names to describe the personality of a candida colony such as star, stipple, smooth, ring, irregular wrinkle, fuzzy, and hat. Each of these is a differently organized microorganism with different survival characteristics.

A fish swims in a sea of water. People live in a sea of microorganisms. We might say it's part of the "Great Plan of Life." Yeast used to be one of the inconsequential inhabitants of the microorganismic sea, but suddenly it is a number-one concern and major threat to our health and quality of life. We must ask the question WHY? Why suddenly is an inconsequential, simple, little, natural inhabitant of the order of things in this world ruining people's lives to the extent candida is?

Before fish were in the sea, there was yeast. Nutritional philosophers speculate that now there may be an attempt by Nature to return to that state and start over again since peoples' life-styles have strayed so far from the laws of Nature and health.

It will do little permanent good to say, "Candida is my enemy. Let's kill candida," because it doesn't tell us WHY it's become our enemy. Killing it alone does not prevent its return: it's only one phase of dealing with this disease. Asking WHY will tell us the cause and, ultimately, the solution. The original title of this discourse was "Candida Is Not Your Enemy." Let's keep our curiosity strong and find out why we have this "new" disease.

First, here is an explanation of the controversial original title, "Candida Is Not Your Enemy". This is a provocative statement if you've ever been acquainted with an environmentally sensitive person whose dysbiosis* has crippled their lives to the extent they've pulled the carpet out of their homes and must wear a gas mask due to their sensitivity to airborn pollutants. But candida is not the enemy. It's only the SYMPTOM of several unnatural facets of our lifestyle. The enemy is whatever suppressed the immune system.

Candida/yeast is everywhere. And it's supposed to be. It's a normal and healthy constituent of the gastrointestinal (G.I.) tract, along with as much as five pounds of various bacteria. It's in the air, in apple cores, in mother's milk, in every breath of air, in the deepest mines, and on the mountain tops.

Candida/yeast, as an inhabitant of the human body, is a parasite. To date no one has found even a symbiotic* relationship between yeast and the human being, so it is generally considered a worthless and benign parasite in its controlled state. Over the course of human existence, a bargain has been struck between the body and the yeast. The bargain is this: Yeast is allowed in the "external" areas of the body and may grow and live in balance with the opposing beneficial bacteria, but may not inhabit the internal body. If it does attempt to colonize in the wrong or undesignated areas, it will be attacked and destroyed by the immune system's white blood cells.

"External" areas include the G.I. (gastrointestinal) tract, vaginal area, nasal area, and the skin. To understand how the G.I. tract is external, you must think of the human body as a donut — with a hole in the middle. From the mouth to the anus there's a pipe in contact with the external environment.

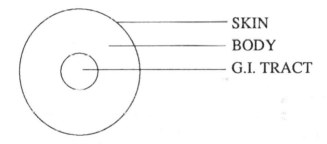

SKIN
BODY
G.I. TRACT

We human beings occupy the apex of life forms on this planet. We're at the top of the planetary food chain and have "dominion" over all the animals. This means that there are no animals that have people as natural, exclusive prey. Whereas the reindeer has the wolf, the mosquito has the frog, the webworm has the wasp, the wildebeest has the lion, and so forth, people are not natural prey. Of course, a person may do in a pinch if they happen to get too close to a hungry lion, tiger, polar bear, or crocodile, but people are not these creatures' natural prey.

But Nature is the great recycler. And the human beings position at the top of the food chain simply means that it's the microorganisms that feed on us.

Philosophers have often made the mistake of viewing the planetary food chain as a linear progression — basically the little fish is eaten by the bigger fish. When they get to human beings, they conjecture that we get to choose what we want to consume and move on into areas of philosophical and spiritual endeavor. But this linear view, in some respects, is in error. Nature recycles and the wheel comes around again, meaning that the guy at the top gets eaten by the guy at the bottom. People are prey to microorganisms by Nature's design.

Shakespeare had the idea when he wrote, "A man may fish with the worm that hath eat of a king, and eat of the fish that hath fed of that worm."

Survival of the Fittest

Another law of Nature comes into play here. The wolf preys on the reindeer — the weakest reindeer. The wolves follow the migrating herds, eating the lame and the sick, thus thinning out the infirm and genetically weak (the runts of the herd). In this fashion they help preserve the strength of the herd as the weak do not live to reproduce and pass on inferior genetic material.

This is the way Nature works. Microorganisms, such as viruses, bacteria, fungi, and parasites, perform the same function with people. When a person is weak or out of balance with Nature, microorganisms increase and cause illness. If a person is constitutionally strong enough to overcome this attack, that person lives. If not, that person dies of infectious disease. This has been the way of Nature since the beginning of time. It's called "survival of the fittest."

From an energy perspective we could say that when a person's oscillations vibrate outside (lower than) the frequency of health, then that person is affected by the microorganisms that inhabit the lower frequency. The result (infection) and counter measure (fever) stimulates the body to return to the realm of healthy oscillations. Viruses are on an even more extreme frequency and cause an even greater healing reaction, or death. While on this subject, researchers of bio-energetic medicine are concerned that genetic engineering experiments with live viruses and monkey liver tissue have created new strains of viruses that can operate more in the human frequency. They cite herpes and the AIDS virus and the body's ineffectiveness to overcome them, as examples.

14

For the microorganisms to flourish, a person must first provide a suitable environment. Poor diet, infectious material penetrating the skin, unsanitary living habits, stressful situations, anger, environmental pollutants, and addictive activities all contribute to the kind of environment microorganisms thrive in. As the microorganisms thrive, the immune system becomes more and more taxed, until it becomes weak, overworked, and either oversensitive or exhausted. A weak immune system means a much less likely ability to survive, for once the immune system is weak, more and more microorganisms take up residence in the body doing what they were designed to do — bring about the demise of the weak.

Having Candidiasis puts people in touch with basic survival, as well as with the basic desire for a good quality of health. For some, it's a strong enough warning that they'll conquer candida no matter what. And a 100% positive attitude is a basic key to survival in any arena.

Antibiotics and Natural Law

A kink was thrown into the normal operation of Nature some fifty years ago with the discovery of antibiotics. By applying antibiotics, medical science was able to stop the microorganisms from performing their function, thus saving countless lives and virtually eliminating the threat of death by infectious disease. Today, tuberculosis, small pox, and syphilis are not the dreaded diseases they were just a few years ago. The natural order has been interrupted. A few doctors today are daring to think that perhaps antibiotics do not thoroughly kill infectious diseases, but only force the body to accept them and end the fight — a conditional surrender rather than a victory. From an energy perspective, antibiotics encourage bacteria to mutate or expand their rate of oscillation. This moves them more into the realm of healthy oscillation, causing more frequent problems — i.e., new varieties with greater activity in the human spectrum. The suppression of bacteria (and the immune system) with antibiotics may have opened the door to the more detrimental viral involvements.

Killing infection, however, does not address the CAUSE. Certainly when your life is on the line you want whatever works. In a life or death situation, no one wants to talk about nutritional philosophy. You just do whatever it takes to survive and do it 100%, now! But the issue here (for times when leisurely discussion is practical) is "why did the microorganisms find a suitable environment for infecting a person?"

There are several answers, one being that the person did not have inherent immunity to that strain of bacteria (such as tetanus from a rusty nail). Another is that the person's immune system was inhibited because the body chemistry was out of balance due to poor nutrition. For example, without proper amino acids to make antibodies, the immune system cannot perform well. Without proper liver function to produce the thousands of needed enzyme systems, the very foundation of life is threatened.

The intervention of antibiotics has saved many a life. Now we are learning it's not without a price. Instead of people dying early of infectious disease, they are now living longer and enjoying it less due to chronic degenerative diseases. People get to live longer now, but in states of cancer, arthritis, osteoporosis, diabetes, and so forth. Only now is the relationship between antibiotics, immunizations (vaccinations), and chronic degenerative diseases being established.

This is not to say that today's medicine is the sole cause of chronic degenerative disease. It's certainly not. Other major considerations are our high acid-ash diets (meat, dairy, refined carbohydrate), improper food combining (using proteins and carbohydrates together in the same meal), pace of life, poor attitudes, stress, and polluted environment. But it all adds up. And candidiasis is right in the middle of it all — the result of going against the natural law.

By intervening in Nature's process, we've intervened and saved the weak reindeer from the wolf's fangs, so to speak. The immune system has been denied its learning experience. And now the global human gene pool is suspected to be inferior to what it used to be, or at least perpetuating a greater amount of weaknesses. (Smoking contributes to this as do a variety of other things.)

This sounds cruel if we say that people should die rather than live to reproduce offspring with inferior immune systems — and this is not what we're saying at all. We're simply looking at how Nature works without bias and without malice. Abide by natural law and flourish. Live outside natural law and have a never-ending struggle to overcome the deep and profound natural processes that work to sustain natural balance.

Antibiotics do not explain why the bacteria got the upper hand with a person, they only come in and kill it indiscriminately. If our treatments were aimed at strengthing the body's natural immune system through natural means such as diet, proper thinking, homeopathics* and herbs, then the body would take care of itself. This is a fundamental difference between the medical approach, which says, "I can kill the bacteria," versus the naturopathic approach, which says, "Let's assist the body naturally to overcome the problem and heal itself." Drugs suppress symptoms. They do not cure.

Candida/fungus will attack the weakest cells. It has an affinity for brains with high aluminum levels (Alzheimer's), joints weakened by amoebas and/or pneumococci (arthritis), livers congested with toxins (allergies), pancreases weakened by sugar and/or small pox vaccinations (diabetes), female systems weakened by birth control pills (premenstrual syndrome, amenorrhea, dysmenorrhea), and so forth.

When I showed a rough draft of some of this material to the famed nutritional researcher, A. Stuart Wheelwright, in November, 1986, he said that I was too easy on matters and only gave part of the picture. He immediately scribbled out a few pages, handed them to me and said, "I'm a little harsh, but I tell it like I see it. You're too easy, so maybe between the two of us we'll hit it just right." Here are Stu's thoughts verbatim.

"Throughout the history of humankind, there have been plagues that scourged the Earth. Candidiasis is the plague of the late 20th century — a penalty we must pay because we have tried to fool with Mother Nature."

"Humanity has scorched the Earth with chemicals in order to produce bigger crops of poorer and poorer food value, then poisoned the body with toxic chemicals in order to keep the weakened flesh working."

"We fail to recognize that good health prevents the invasion of disease. The law of Nature states, 'Only the fit survive.' The unfit perish. We have bread to feed an unfit world. We have kept the weakened and innately sick artificially alive, so they have procreated and brought forth more of their kind. The hardy people have been inundated with chemical medicines that have destroyed their natural strength and they have become weak. The weak have been

17

synthetically stimulated to reach a degree of normalcy through further drugging."

"The chemicals of our society by their very nature can never build health. They stimulate or sedate the various organs, tissues, and glands. A drug by its structure never builds life, but may give a stimulus to make the body feel good. The individual moves from one stimulus to another."

"On awakening in the morning, the average person in the U.S. will reach for a cup of coffee. In most instances the coffee-stimulant was not strong enough, so ways were developed to make it more and more stimulating — from drip to percolated to cappuccino [expresso]. Then during the day there are colas, none of which build vitality or good body tissue. For breakfast there's dry cereal or instantized, processed cereals that have few life support factors and homo milk that damages the blood vessels. Then lunch is a sandwich or hamburger made from meat that may be three months old from cattle laced with steroids and other chemicals to make them grow fast. Should a person drink tap water, it includes 35 added chemicals plus the industrial and agricultural residues (which are almost totally free of natural, organic material so essential to healthy vegetables) used to stimulate the production of vegetables from worn out soil."

"Some crops are sprayed weekly during their growth, and what doesn't cover the plant most surely gets into the soil. The ammonia used to stimulate vegetable growth leaves a residue in the soil that must eventually be neutralized with other chemicals. The potassium and phosphorus comes from chemicals, not natural sources, and also upsets the potentials of the soil."

"Fruits are grown in orchards plumbed with chemical spray systems, so the farmer merely pushes a button and the trees are doused with poisons and the fruit produced is permeated to the core with them."

"Every few years the poisons must be made stronger and stronger because the bugs keep getting stronger and stronger to resist the poisons. The same is true of antibiotics and the bacteria they aim to kill."

"In our bodies, the doping and drugging keep breeding stronger, more resistant strains of bacteria, viruses, fungi, parasites, and crystals, so new and more poisonous drugs must be produced to kill them. And our bodies do not build greater and greater resistances because a bug or germ goes through numerous cycles of creation. We have to contend with new and more virulent diseases every few years — diseases that progress faster than our immune systems can catch up to them."

"Back 30 years ago there were a few cases of candidiasis — perhaps one to three per hundred and something, but it was not so virulent and destructive as it is now. Today we find candidiasis in 90 percent of the people tested in northern California by Dr. Clary in his recent research report. I find it in 60 to 70 percent of the people in Texas, Arizona, and Florida."

"Dr. Clary says that it's no longer an epidemic: it's a pandemic*. And he thinks when the nation finally realizes what's happening there will be pandemonium. A doctor in Dallas told me that at least half the deaths now are directly or indirectly related to candida or related fungus. The reports do not show this, but fungus was the cause even though other complications are what the death was attributed to."

"A disease that is caused by medicine and drugging cannot be cured by medicine and drugging."

"Candidiasis is a doctor-induced, drug-produced disease that causes destruction of the immune system. Yeast overgrowth is the result, and candidiasis is the result of yeast overgrowth. The medical doctors attribute the cause to antibiotics, the anti-fertility pill, and anti-inflammatory steroids. I suspect that the drugs being used to treat candidiasis only push it deeper into the tissues and make it more difficult to deal with when it resurfaces. Time will tell."

After jotting that down on a piece of scratch paper, Wheelwright left Texas for his lab in Utah to continue his research for nutritional answers to candidiasis.

Rather than more and more attempts to outsmart Nature and cover up our mistakes, the question should be, "How can we live in accord with natural law?" rather than, "How can we beat the system?" And this doesn't mean a "back-to-nature movement" where people have to give up plumbing, central heating, and video recorders. We're referring to an evolution that works with Nature rather than against it. Human ego wants to master weather and control it. Human wisdom would choose to work along with it, to reach an agreement. The relationship is similar to a horse that can't be broken, yet it can be ridden by a rider who establishes an understanding based on respect.

Following natural law, medicine should seek to support and enhance the body's own immune systems, rather than intervening and imposing a narrow-sighted reaction.

Natural law is both exacting and flexible. If we cut down a tree to make paper, perhaps that tree should be replaced. The global impact of the stripping of the Amazon jungle (5000 acres a day) means less oxygen is being replenished. Combine this with what we are dumping into the atmosphere from industry and transportation, and a major problem is already underway. Could there be a way of farming in the Amazon whereby the jungle could reclaim the land — working with Nature rather than against it? Could a factory provide oxygen mechanically? Should greenbelts be maintained? We have the ability to enjoy the fruits of the Earth without creating severe imbalances — ones that Nature will dispassionately seek to re-balance on all levels.

The human body has very efficient and exceedingly complex systems to maintain balance and the pH (alkalinity) of the blood. So does Nature on the global scale.

Nature provides answers to health concerns more in accord with it's laws, unlike the intervention of drugs, and that allows a person to survive infection and end up with a healthier immune system! [This is discussed in the section on herbal answers to bacteria, viruses, and fungi.]

It is the dream of naturopaths like myself that one day our incredible medical sciences with their great research, technology, and skilled, dedicated physicians will embrace the validity of the natural laws that govern health and bring forth true and whole healing of the human body. This will involve a much greater understanding of the energies of the body (electro-acupuncture, homeopathy) and the prudent use of herbs - living medicines for a living body.

The point to understand is that drugs are only one way to get results. The impact of "dead" chemical drugs on the human biosystem are quite profound. They cause changes, but do not cure. While helping one area of the body, they usually damage another. Hence the frightening side effects of drugs as listed in the Physicians' Desk Reference. Drugs are very exacting. They can only stimulate or sedate and do so with precision. That's one of the major reasons we've adopted them into our society. Since they are so exacting and able to manifest the same results time after time, what makes people think that they are immune to all the side effects? Ignorance and blind trust in science are two possible answers.

Drugs such as antibiotics interfere with the body's learning processes. If every time a body has a sore throat (an early warning that it's out of step with natural law) an antibiotic is given to kill the bacteria, the body never learns what it is to be a winner — to be victorious in its fight against an invader. The big brother antibiotic took care of the situation, denying the body the experience and the memory of how to fight again if needed.

Yes, the sore throat is gone, but the body has not learned much or completed its natural cleansing cycles. And even worse, the body may have accepted the bacteria and in the future will not put up much of a fight. Where there is no fight, there is no fever and soreness, and thus the appearance of being well when the real state is much less than optimal.

With biological medicines such as homeopathy, the remedies stimulate the natural immune response and compress the time line (the duration of the illness) so the body responds quickly and thoroughly, and completes its natural cycle becoming the self-educated victor.

The results are often faster than drug therapy in many acute conditions such as ear infections, sore throat, headaches, and so forth.

Some statistics: Approximately 3/4 of the world's population does NOT use drugs, but relies on herbs for healing. 7/8 of these "primitive" nations are healthier than the people of the United States, according to the United Nations survey. Of course, there are other factors involved, such as diet and climate, but medicine has ment in longevity is evident, but that is a result of fewer infant deaths, and not a sign of better health.

For instance, in both kinesiology (muscle testing) and electro-acupuncture (measurement of electrical resistance in the body's meridian system), chemical heart medication tests to be beneficial to a person with heart problems. But it also tests to damage the liver and kidneys. Drugs give with one hand and take with the other. But herb-based formulas (derived from living ingredients, such as plants, nutriments, and protomorphagens*), designed to support the natural processes of the heart nutritionally, test to help the heart as well as support the whole body systemically. And this is a fundamental difference between allopathic (drug-oriented) medicine and biological (homeopathic*, naturopathic) medicine.

When a person waits so long to remedy an ailment that it becomes a disease, drastic medicines are often needed just to preserve the life. But if a person learns to correct stresses before they threaten life, then natural means are much more viable. This is why health evaluation methods such as sclerology, kinesiology, electro-acupuncture, and to some extent iridology, are so valuable. Catch the problem before it develops and biological medicines provide ready answers often more swiftly and effectively than drugs,without the side effects and dangers!

So candida's role in the order of things is a benign yeast whose job is to ferment sugars and perhaps, when dead, it might even become a usable nutrient to the body. But with our unnatural diet, unnatural medicines, unnatural stresses on our immune system, and unnatural environment, we cause unnatural behavior in this simple, single-cell plant thatis now wreaking havoc of pandemic proportions in people's lives.

CANDIDA AND NUTRITIONAL YEAST

Over the last 40 years in the health movement, nutritional yeast has been considered a wonder food by many health-promoters, a highly nutritious food source rich in B-vitamins, DNA/RNA, chromatin factors, trace minerals, and available amino acids. Health food stores sell tons of nutritional yeast as a dietary supplement each week. These are called such names as brewer's yeast (from beer), debittered yeast (from beer, but cleaned of beer residues), torula yeast (from the paper industry), and engovita yeast (from molasses).

Occasionally a nutritional leader would cite yeast as a high stress food, difficult to digest, primarily because of its high carbohydrate to protein values. So yeast has not been without controversy, even before candida became an issue.

An assay of its nutritional qualities shows it to be very rich in nutriments. But this is not the only criterion for eating something. Bio-availability is an even more important factor. Can the body assimilate and utilize the nutriments? Commercial yeast supplements do not rate very high on the bio-force scale. The body has some difficulty utilizing its riches. However, it is a very suitable food for cats and dogs, as they have a stronger hydrochloric acid content in their stomachs and can digest and utilize the tougher parts of yeast-protein.

There are still some misconceptions about commercial yeast. There is a fundamental difference between candida yeast and nutritional yeast — one is living and one is dead. Candida yeast is a viable, living yeast, as is baker's yeast, that is capable of reproducing in the body environment. It's major role in life is to ferment sugars, be fruitful, and multiply. Nutritional yeast is usually a non-viable, dead yeast rich in nutrients such as B vitamins, amino acids, and nucleic acids. People are not allergic to the action of nutritional yeast, because there is none — it's non-viable. But they may be sensitive to nutritional yeast in the same way a person can be sensitive to beef, corn, dairy, wheat, shellfish, broccoli, avocados, and so forth. And there are some other considerations that we will discuss.

People with candidiasis are sensitive to almost all viable yeasts and most likely quite sensitive to non-viable yeasts like nutritional yeast.

When candidiasis is present, people become sensitive to yeast, fungi, and molds. It seems that organisms similar to yeast-fungus triggers an immune response, whether they are yeast in foods, mushrooms, musty cellars, airborne molds, or moldy leaves in the yard. This sensitivity taxes the immune system (causes overreaction initially, lethargic response later) and by doing so supports the proliferation of the detrimental form of yeast — the fungal form. Also, poor digestion of nutritional yeasts creates allergenic amino acids and toxins due to fermentation, and people with candidiasis invariably have poor digestion.

This sensitivity forms the basis for the severely limiting "Candida Diets" that eliminate all sugars, molds, yeasts, fungi, and suspected allergins from the diet. But before weeping in despair, new insights regarding diet will be forthcoming in this material that will show that a terribly restrictive diet may NOT be necessary!

Another reason for restricting nutritional yeast when candidiasis is present is the significant estradiol (female hormone estrogen) content. Candida and several other varieties of fungi flourish in the presence of estrogen (and testosterone — male hormone).

This is one of several reasons many nutritionists take a stand against birth control pills and excessive use of hormones given after hysterectomies. That is in addition to a strong objection to the operation itself.

There is a strong correlation between the endocrine gland system and cellular immunity. Hormones perform a function that also causes a chain reaction from other glands. There is a complex system of feedback loops, and biologists and endocrinologists have only begun to fathom the implications. Glands support and contradict each other. They help and oppose each other's actions in accordance with an inherent system of balance yet to be fully understood. The adrenal gland is part of our immune system, yet it can act in opposition to the thymus gland — the heart of the immune system — when stressed. The message here is that when we interfere with the endocrine system, many diseases and conditions manifest, such as diabetes, candidiasis, osteoporosis, P.M.S., hypoglycemia, etc. Birth control pills interfere with the whole body's endocrine system.

Estrogen is known to be essential for calcium utilization, feminine characteristics, and mental stability. It is also known to weaken cellular immunity, contribute to breast cancer, promote yeast growth, and impair oxygen absorption. Many people think that, because it is such a two-edged sword, estrogen regulation would be better left to the body's natural wisdom and not be used to achieve infertility. There are other effective birth control methods that do not systemically harm the body. The new cervical cap tested in Austin, Texas, by the Austin Women's Self-Help Group which is now fully approved and provided by Planned Parenthood is a good example.

So nutritional yeast, although it is non-viable, still contains elements that can hinder recovery from excessive yeast/fungus proliferation.

If a person is not bothered with candida and has a strong digestive system (adequate hydrochloric acid production in the stomach), then nutritional yeast might remain something of a food supplement. Another concern regarding yeast supplementation is that, if eaten alone, it probably won't be properly digested. Since yeast is a powder and doesn't have much substance, the stomach will pass it along very quickly — too soon for the proteins to be broken down. It is easy for yeast to putrify in the intestine and thus contribute to the stress of the body. This is the case where yeast or yeast-containing protein powders are drunk with fruit juice. The complex proteins do not mix properly with digestive acids and thus do not digest properly.

People with candidiasis must be careful until such a time that their digestion, intestinal flora, and immune systems are strong again. And since so few people have successfully recovered from candidiasis, we really don't know if strong viable-yeast-based foods (breads, apple cider vinegar, soy sauce, beer, etc.) will ever be on the menu again. In theory they should, but most theories are based on the concept of the body without taking into consideration such factors as air and water pollution, agricultural soil-nutrient depletion, and the myriad chemicals put in foods all which test and stress the immune system.

25

The real issues are whether or not the immune system overreacts to yeast foods, and if the foods cause yeast proliferation. The best advice is to avoid yeasty foods if candidiasis is a concern.

There is a yeast form that most candidiasis patients can use in small amounts such as are found in a few high quality supplements. I know this sounds contrary to what the books say, but few authors have really looked into the matter. It's called AUTOLYZED YEAST. It is totally predigested into its elemental parts. Autolyzed yeast is in some of the higher quality nutritional supplements to provide B vitamins, trace elements, and chromatin (genetic) factors. Such nutritional formulas test surprisingly well for people with candidiasis. Evidently, whatever the allergin factor in yeast is, the autolization process seems to render it unrecognizable. The point here is hard-and-fast rules regarding human nutrition often have exceptions.

The product label should read "autolyzed yeast," not just "yeast," or "nutritional yeast," which may be quite reactive. So check the label. If in doubt, seek a non-yeast source.

DR. JEKYLL AND MR. HYDE — THE TWO FACES OF CANDIDA ALBICANS

As we've learned, candida albicans is a yeast that naturally inhabits the G.I. tract in a symbiotic relationship with the other constituents of the intestinal flora. The difficulty begins when it overpopulates, particularly in a biotin (a B vitamin) deficient environment, because then it changes both its physiology and anatomy and becomes a cell-invasive, parasitic fungus that seeks to destroy the body.

This means that this "simple" yeast is really quite complex. Trillions of strains are genetically possible, so candida is readily adaptable and a formidable opponent to the human immune system.

If the environment (temperature and food supply) were optimal, yeast could take over the world. We would not have oceans of water; we'd have oceans (and mountains) of yeast. Since yeast reproduces in geometric proportions, one minute there can be a thousand yeast cells and the next minute there can be a billion. The thing that keeps planet Earth from being one giant yeast colony is environment. Temperatures vary, and food supply (sugars, carbohydrates) are not available enough to support such a population.

Our G.I. tracts provide a wonderful environment for yeast — constant temperature, moist atmosphere. What about food source? Many people have a fairly constant supply of sugar and carbohydrates (bread) coming through the tubes to keep large colonies of yeast in candy-shop paradise.

Once candida/fungus colonizes and takes up residence in an area, produces toxins as a by-product of its cellular activity. This further stresses the body as it must now deal with these toxins. When the fungus dies of old age, the body must dispose of the remains, which are also quite toxic.

The toxins damage other areas of the body (brain, kidneys, liver) and account for many of the symptoms of depression, food allergies, spaceyness, and forgetfulness. These toxins are antigenic* (cause immune reactions) and weaken the immune system.

In 1981, seventy-nine antigen-toxins were identified to result from yeast. By 1986, over 200 were identified. In 1987 the official number is 257 toxins, and each one can cause different symptoms in different individuals. Some interfere with the metabolism of sugar, others interfere with the hormonal system, and others interfere with the neurotransmitters in the brain.

When people talk about candida "die-off," they are referring to the poisoning of the body with dead fungus. Eventually the toxic dead fungus is carried out of the body through the kidneys and the colon, but as long as it's in the body, people can feel effects such as fatigue, headaches, and depression. In homeopathy and in the nutritional sciences this is often referred to as an "aggravation,"or a "side show, " and the illness flares up, apparently worse, during the cleansing process.

One of the myths of both homeopathic and nutritional therapies is that the body must go into a healing crisis to restore health. More often such reactions are signs that the therapy is working too fast and pushing too hard and a little wear and tear can be avoided by going easier on the program or by providing more detoxification (colon and kidney) support. This may be as simple as increasing water, increasing vitamin C, or using herbal chelators. In every case, cleansings are an individual matter.

It is important to realize that for some people the evidence that their anti-candida program is working is that they temporarily feel even worse. Should this occur, they should reduce the dosages of their program, drink additional water, and move the bowels (with a hydragogue laxative such as oxygenated cascara sagrada and aloe, rather than irritating laxatives, like most drug store varieties, senna, magnesium, and so forth). A day or two later they will be able to resume the program, usually with noticeable improvement.

Candida albicans is dimorphic, meaning it's a shape-changer. The yeast state is non-invasive. It's content to live in the G.I. tract and vaginal area and ferment sugars all the livelong day. But in overpopulation or in a biotin-deficient environment, it sends out mercenaries in an invasive, fungal form. This fungal form of candida is the troublemaker. It grows rhizoids (tentacles) that penetrate cells and destroys them. Here's where the trouble begins.

Too much yeast is a problem (as in thrush or vaginal infec-

28

tions), but when it changes to a fungus it becomes pathogenic*. Candida's ability to change gives it a survival factor that makes it difficult to eliminate. It waxes and wanes with cycles of its own. If attacked, it can change its shape (DNA) and avoid being killed. This is why some researchers think the drug Nystatin is creating new and more virulent strains of candida in the same way antibiotics are responsible for stronger strains of bacteria.

The fungus disease, candidiasis, invades and destroys the mucosa or protective lining of the intestines. This mucosa is important as a protection to the G.I. tract and it plays a vital role in the absorption of nutrients. When there's a breakdown of the mucosa, there is a two-fold problem created.

One problem with a damaged mucosa is that partially-digested foods can enter the bloodstream — particularly proteins. These food particles are recognized by the immune system as antigens*, which cause allergic reactions — enemies to fight. This sends the immune system into Red Alert, and it must work to fight these antigenic nutrients that are now in the wrong place at the wrong time and have become enemies. The result is that the immune system becomes exhausted because it is stimulated so frequently.

In the past, it was thought by medical science that the G.I. tract would not allow the absorption of large, unusable molecules. This is a new idea. W. Allen Walker, M.D., pediatric gastrointestinal specialist at Massachusetts General Hospital writes in "Gastroenterology, 1974":

"The normal adult gastrointestinal tract is assumed to be an impermeable and impenetrable barrier to the uptake and transport of macromolecules. This concept is supported by the fact that intraluminal digestive processes are available to efficiently break down large molecular weight substances and therefore minimize macromolecular contact with the mucosal surface. Furthermore, no known mechanism has been described for the transport of macromolecules from the intestinal lumen across the gut wall into the circulation. Despite this popular notion, there is increasing evidence that the normal adult intestine is in fact permeable to macromolecules, not in sufficient quantities to be of nutritional importance, but in quantities that may be antigenic or biologically active. This observation could mean quantities of bacteria, endotoxin, proteolytic and hydrolytic enzymes, or of ingested antigens that normally exist in the intestinal lumen and therefore might be of considerable importance in the pathogenesis of a number of local intestinal and systemic disease states."

Here we have the basis for the belief in the absorption of allergins, and yeast itself, into the bloodstream — one way to explain the many symptoms of candidiasis.

The November, 1984, issue of *The Lancet* presented a study linking the use of aspirin with increased intestinal permeability. The eight authors summarized their research saying "the administration of NSAIDS (non-steroidal anti-inflammatory drugs, i.e., aspirin) may lead to loss of intestinal integrity, thus facilitating antigen absorption and perhaps contributing to the persistence of the disease."

Millions of aspirins are eaten daily. Could this be contributing to the widespread intestinal malfunctions, allergies, and food sensitivities so prevalent today? Nutritionists have known for years that aspirin causes the stomach to bleed a little. And now the TV tells us to take aspirin to prevent heart attacks. [The initial research on aspirin and heart attacks was conducted in England with something like Alka-Seltzer and aspirin with alkaline buffers. No one thought to investigate the alkalizing factors. They may have a bearing on body pH, which is known to affect the heart muscle.]

It is common for people with candidiasis to be sensitive to foods and the environment. Allergic reactions to anything getting into the bloodstream before it's properly digested are quite common. Some incompletely digested proteins can cause severe mood swings and altered mental states, including depression, memory loss, and extreme behaviors.

Through the bloodstream, these toxins can reach the brain and interfere with the receptors, nerve impulses, memory, and behavior patterns. The toxins are labeled "exorphins," meaning they come from outside the body, as opposed to "endorphins," which act on the receptors to control many biochemical aspects of health such as pain control. Exorphins are irritants and cause many allergic symptoms including asthma, hives, heart palpitations, and deep tissue pain.

On the other hand, in certain instances candidiasis may block the assimilation of vital amino acids causing malabsorption syndrome. Amino acids such as taurine, tyrosine, tryptophan, and arginine may be hindered at the intestinal mucosa (lining) if it's inundated with candida.

Also, since the beneficial lactobacillus is lacking, the nutrients provided to the body by its fermentation processes are also lacking. We already know that a lack of biotin provides a suitable environment for candidiasis. Nutrients related to the presence of beneficial bacteria include a number of B vitamins such as pantothenic acid, folic acid, niacin (B-3), biotin, riboflavin (B-2), pyridoxine (B-6), and B-12.

If the intestinal wall is clogged up with candida, nutrient absorption can be inhibited. If the mucosa is damaged, improperly digested materials may be absorbed into the bloodstream as antigens.

The other problem a candida-damaged mucosa causes is that the fungus itself gets into the blood stream and must also be fought by the immune system. If the immune system is overtaxed, or rather WHEN the immune system gets overtaxed, the candida fungus is able to leave the bloodstream and invade tissue. It is not uncommon to find candida colonies in the brain, pancreas, liver, kidneys, and deep tissue such as hips, in people plagued by chronic candidiasis. Since most of the drug and nutritional therapies only work in the G.I. tract and vaginal areas, deep-tissue candidiasis is much more difficult to remedy. But nutrition has answers for this too, as we'll soon see.

SYSTEMIC CANDIDIASIS AND ITS SYMPTOMS

Now that we're more familiar with yeast and some of the basic issues of candida, but before we delve into the specific causes, let's look a little more thoroughly at the symptoms of candida.

Candida, when it is localized to just one area of the body such as the colon or vagina, presents a relatively simple problem of contained overgrowth. By reducing the amount of yeast (by whatever method) the body is able to reestablish its own controls.

When, through constant exposure, the immune system chooses to not respond to the presence of yeast/fungus, the problem becomes systemic with candida-involvement occuring in many different places — usually areas weakened from a variety of causes (toxic metals, injury, genetic weakness, exposure to chemical toxins, etc.)

Candidiasis involvement can effect specific body systems to the point where there is a clear enough picture to suspect the damaging effects of candida. Whenever candida involvement goes beyond a localized infection, it is actually affecting the whole body. None of the body systems work independently of each other. Candida can not affect one body system without affecting the whole body in some way.

Let's take a look a several body systems and how candida can be a disruptive factor. Keep in mind that candida in a body system may not be the ultimate cause of ill-health in that system, but its presence causes further destruction and more symptoms, and therefore correcting the Candidiasis can bring massive relief and the opportunity for the immune system to be better able to respond to the real challenge.

Allergic Response of the Immune System

Allergic reactions are an "altered reactivity" of the immune system and can include reactions such as headaches, runny nose, asthma, hives, depression, hypoglycemia, irritability, arthritis, etc. which do not affect other people in similiar conditions.

People who have allergies are susceptable to Candidiasis and people with Candidiasis are prone to developing allergies. The allregic reaction is a hyper (overactive) immune response. Candidiasis is a hypo (underactive or suppressed) immune response. Any imbalance or stress to the immune system can allow candida proliferation. Candida itself introduces antigenic toxins which weaken the immune system and cause allergenic responses. This "chicken or the egg" situation is important to understand because in some people, both candida and allergies must be treated at the same time to have success. Both the hyper and hypo aspects of the immune system must be brought into balance.

Martha, a 45-year-old hispanic lady had been on allergy shots and antihistamines for three years, yet every change in airborne pollens brought a new bout of headaches and wheezing. Overweight, lethargic, and depressed were here self-assigned characteristics.

In June, 1987 she began a comprehensive candida program with additional supports for the liver and endocrine glands (thyroid, adrenals). After an initial die off reaction which was surprisingly mild, her allergic symptoms improved dramatically in only two weeks. She embraced the Pro-Vita!*Plan* and during the next three months she lost 22 pounds and only experienced two headaches which were milder than before and no wheezing occurred.

Her allergist allowed her to stop the allergy injections and she began an anti-candida maintenance program. By December she had lost 41 pounds and was virtually a new person.

The advent of the cedar season knocked her for a loop and she virtually fell apart with a massive histamine reaction (runny nose, burning eyes, dizzy.) But the apparent set back was quickly corrected with herbal antifungal factors and a 5x potentization of monilia albicans (candida). She did not respond to potentized cedar or juniper.

We learned conclusively in December that candida was the predisposing factor in her allergies.

1988 was dedicated to natural therapies to strengthen the immune system, build the endocrine system, cleanse and rebuild the liver in alternating months with a month of rest (no therapies) in between. By December 1988, the now trim and viviacious Martha went through cedar season with only a twinge of discomfort — one which corresponded to New Year's Eve celebrations.

It is reasonable to suspect that the gradual weakening of the immune system over the years due to her frequent antibiotic use and the subsequent increase of candida involvement contributed directly to her gradual increase of allergies which were finally identified by her doctor and treated with allergy shots. Only when she was able to master candida AND rebuild the affected body systems was she able to hold her own, without medications, in a more optimal state of health.

Gastro-Intestinal System (G.I. Tract) Symptoms

Digestion/elimination is one of the most predominant areas of Candidiasis symptoms — gas, bloating, gastritis, ulcers, heartburn all relate to the upper G.I. tract; food allergies, sugar cravings for the middle G.I. tract; and diarrhea, constipation, flatulence, inflammations, anal rashes are common for the lower G.I. tract.

The G.I. tract will be disscussed in detail throughout this book, but basically once candida is able to increase in the G.I. tract, the eating of sugars and refined carbohydrates feeds the yeast and causes it to multiply causing gas and bloating form the carbon dioxide released from its fermentation processes.

If the candida yeast invades the intestinal mucosa, food particles can be absorbed before they are sufficiently digested causing food allergies.

Candida/yeast causes increased prostaglandin production — an anti-inflammatory chemical — which can result in constipation, diarrhea, or an alternation of these symptoms. In the "American Journal of Physiology 1984, Dr. Sanders reports, "yeast induced prostaglandins released by various tissues of the G.I. tract may produce gastro esophageal sphincter relaxation and increased intragastric pressure which could contribute to esophageal reflux."

This means candida can make a person burp up. But it shows how a symptom such as acid reflux can be caused by candida in the G.I. tract.

This can be a serious problem in that should a person burp up stomach acids during sleep, the acids can burn the cardiac valve which holds the food down in the stomach. Weakening the valve means that stomach acids can chronically burp up into the mouth during sleep and destroy tooth enamel. This has actually happened.

People have lost their teeth due to acid reflux. Such people have to sleep sitting up to avoid further damage.

Cardiovascular System Symptoms

In the preceeding "Allergic Response of the Immune System" section we showed how the endocrine and hepatic (liver) systems were also involved. With the Cardiovascular system, the immune, endocrine and hepatic systems are also involved as well as the urinary and lymphatic systems.

A basic tenet of naturopathic healing is that the whole body is interrelated to each of its parts meaning if you affect one part, you also affect the whole or all the other parts.

In a healthy body, yeast/fungus (should it ever find its way into the blood stream) would not last long as antibodies would bind it and the immune system would kill it. But with a suppressed immune response, yeast/fungus can move through the blood stream and infect other areas. Candida can feed on red blood cells.

Furthermore, toxins from dead candida can cause allergic reactions and affect mood (depression), cause dizziness, and fluid retention (edema).

Although Candidiasis is not a cardiovascular disease, its effects can cause heart palpitations, irregular heart beat, and racing heart spells due to its interference with the endocrine hormones and allergenic responses of the immune system.

A quick example is Roy, an athletic doctor of chiropractic with symptoms of occasional bouts of rapid pulse and anxiety. His history includes taking every nutritional supplement for the heart he could find. Nutritional therapy (Pro-Vita! Plan) and naturopathic therapy for Candidiasis quickly put an end to this condition along with a host of other previously-not-discussed digestive complaints.

Genito-Urinary System Symptoms

Vaginal yeast infections and yeast related bladder infections, PMS, diaper rash, urethritis, bed wetting, chronic prostate difficulties, and genital rashes can all be the result of candida involvement.

Oftentimes people wish to think of vaginal yeast as a localized problem, not a systemic one. While at the onset this may be true, and while topical applications of remedies can end an episode, clinical experience has taught that systemic treatment is necessary. This is in accord with the wholistic view of health. The whole body needs a strengthening against the proliferation of yeast, not just the vaginal area alone.

And one step further regarding the nursing infant with thrush, diaper rash, vaginal discharge, etc., the mother should undertake energetic-based natural therapy as well as the baby.

For men, candida has become a new area to investigate regarding solutions to chronic prostate problems. Candida can be passed back and forth during sexual intercourse. Should candida take up residence in the prostate, many urinary and sexual-function problems can occur such as dribbling, burning urination, lack of urinary pressure, premature ejaculation, as well as chronic allergies (sinusitis).

Respiratory System Symptoms

Since yeast is in every breath of air, respiratory involvement with Candidiasis is quite common. Symptoms such as asthma, sore throat, canker sores, chronic cough, thrush, sinus infections, pneumonia, bronchitis, etc. are all linked with Candidiasis.

Endocrine System Symptoms

The hormonal system is profoundly affected by candida resulting in PMS, chronic fatigue, depression, apathy, confusion, allergies, hypoglycemia, etc. It is suspected that candida and its toxins interfere with the hormonal communications resulting in a misfiring or out-of-synch condition.

Candida prefers some hormones as a food source and prevents them from entering the cells and accomplishing their mission. Since the endocrine system is dependent on hormonal messengers to turn itself on and off, candida disrupts its communications by interfering with the hormones.

Muscular System Symptoms

Chiropractors are becoming very aware of candida involvement with their patients whose adjustments fail to "hold." Weakness, charley horses, deep muscle pains in the neck and shoulders, poor coordination, bumping into things, fibromyalgia can all be a result of candida's effects on the muscles. Candida can actually inhabit the muscles and inhibit proper nourishment of muscle tissue as well as proper elimination of metabolic wastes. Muscular stress can cause spinal misalignment and nerve impingement.

Nervous System Symptoms

Candida affects the nervous system via the endocrine hromones and muscular system. If the hormonal system is out of sync, the hypothalmus portion of the brain is stressed. The hypothalmus serves as a switchboard or center of communication. If "calls" are being misrouted, then the body's metabolism is altered. Stress hormones released by tissues in the presence of candida become irritants to the nerves resulting in headaches, migraines, anxiety, irritability, and even hypoglycemia. Candida joins the ranks of the herpes virus as a nerve-related problem.

Communication is vitally important in any arena, and is certainly of paramount importance to the body. If communication is disrupted, very little can work. Candidiasis disrupts the body's communication system.

Summary of System Symptoms

We could present a scenario for candida disrupting every body system and the profound effects it has on the whole person. Something that is so disruptive creates a wide and complex variety of symptoms, none of which are completely unique to Candidiasis. By looking deeper into this issue, we'll learn how to protect ourselves from the micro-organisms in our environment.

Subcutaneous Candida Incubation

One fact often overlooked is that candida can incubate under the skin. There is not much research directed in this area. The skin is a much-neglected area among nutritional researchers even though it is the body's second-largest organ and has a profound effect on other organs.

Candida under the skin is called subcutaneous candida. Evidence points to the use of alkaline soap as a primary cause.

It has long been known that soap encourages the growth of bacteria. Being alkaline, it disrupts the natural acid mantle of the skin and provides a soap scum medium on which bacteria proliferate. Furthermore, the antibacterial soaps (deodorant soaps) kill the beneficial flora of the skin, creating the same effect that antibiotics cause in the G.I. tract — an ideal environment for candidiasis.

In the subcutaneous tissue, particles of alkali soap scum may form breeding grounds for candida colonization. It is important to realize that focusing on the G.I. tract is not enough to conquer candida. A whole body approach is needed.

Once again, it's herbology to the rescue. There are herbal "soaps" that contain no soap, but use yucca, white amid bark, sweet birch, etc., with natural sudsing agents (hydroxypropyl methylcellulose - the outer layer of sea kelp) and natural anti-candida factors. These make excellent shampoos, body soaps, face soaps, and skin care products that do not damage the skin. They are completely free of chemicals. Clinically this is significant.

The herb echinacea stimulates the immune system temporarily (until homeostasis renders it ineffective in about 10-14 days) and can be used in short cycles to improve the body's immune response.

Homeopathic potentizations of the mineral silica (silicea) prove to increase macrophage (immune system's house cleaners) activity.

Oxygen increases lymphocyte viability, so the mineral germanium, as well as stabilized oxygen (not hydrogen peroxide), are promising immune assistants.

Candida on the skin means that the virulent forms can be transmitted sexually, so candidiasis is now an infectious venereal disease. Vaginal and prostate-based candidiasis can continue to affect the whole system regardless of what is done to fight candida in the G.I. tract.

Candida/fungus feeds on blood cells and nerves. It literally eats the body alive.

Candida proliferation and a weak immune system go hand in hand. This is why it is so critically important to conquer candida and rebuild the immune system in order to enjoy a healthful life.

Candidiasis is an iatrogenic (doctor-induced) disease, for the most part. It existed prior to antibiotics, but now that allopathic medicine is at its pinnacle, candidiasis has become rampant. And so far, doctors are having trouble curing this disease, as can be seen by the number of people who've been on and off nystatin — the drug of choice for candidiasis — for years and still have problems with yeast. Perhaps it's time to look to nutrition for answers — where some quite remarkable answers are being found today!

CANDIDA AND THE IMMUNE SYSTEM

The body's immune system is responsible for defending against yeast invasion in any form. Should any yeast or fungus get into the bloodstream, the immune system's forces are supposed to clean it up. But what if the immune system is weak or handicapped? Then the fungus continues in the bloodstream and can soon invade tissues.

Immune system deficiencies are becoming more and more prevalent. Many think this is due to the same reasons candida is such a widespread disease — use of drugs, antibiotics, immunizations, poor diet, silver amalgam dental fillings, use of addictive substances (caffeine, tobacco, sugar), lack of full spectrum light, lack of exercise, chemical preservatives, pesticides, and higher stress levels.

Vaccinations

People often ask, "Aren't vaccinations (immunizations) supposed to strengthen the immune system?" This is a subject covered in depth in other publications, but basically immunizations provide the disease, or pieces of the disease, to the immune system so it can fight it and remember how to quickly construct antibodies to the disease should it ever encounter it again.

Doctors and nutritionists against vaccinations believe that oftentimes the live virus that is introduced into the body as a vaccine continues to live in the body in a "cold war" or smoldering state. There is strong evidence that the cowpox vaccine for smallpox can nest in the pancreas and lead to diabetes over the years. And even if a person did not have a smallpox vaccination, but one of the parents did, that person can inherit a weakness (known as a "miasm" in homeopathy) and have a tendency toward pancreatic disorders.

Pancreas disorders contribute to high blood sugar (the liver and adrenal glands are also involved), which provides an abundant food source to candida. For this reason, diabetics have a particulary difficult time with candida.

The progressive medical doctors in Europe often give an

immunization with the biological antidote (homeopathic nosode*) in the same injection, because they want to be sure the body throws off and drains out the toxic virus (or material) being injected in the vaccine. The nosode is a 30x potentization of the disease, to the point where there is no physical substance left — only the freed oscillations or energy pattern of the disease. The energy patterns cause release of the disease from the tissue so it can be eliminated via the immune system.

Why this is not understood very well is modern science is only acquainted with the chemical nature of the immune system — not the electrical or bio-energetic nature. The body is primarily an electrical or wave form system and so is the immune system. The chemistry system is a subset of this energetic system.

The case against vaccinations began many years ago, but has been actively suppressed by the American Medical Association and by various government agencies, which have gone so far as to ban books and forcibly remove them from health food stores. (Land of the free?) It is once again becoming an issue as, now, maverick medical doctors are reporting that oftentimes more people have adverse reactions or die from reactions to vaccines than is acceptable by even the medical profession's liberal standards, though we seldom hear about it. The infamous swine flu vaccine debacle a few years ago is a good example.

Some candidiasis-alerted medical doctors attempt to vaccinate against candida with a program called "desensitization," whereby live candida is injected under the skin. This is examined in the "Treatment" section, but results are not particularly promising.

Some researchers speculate that the body does not thoroughly overcome virulent infections, but ends up accepting them thus calling a truce and no longer reacting to them. People seem well, but the disease smolders, weakening the entire immune system over the years. This is sometimes seen in elderly people who seem to be in excellent health until some trauma occurs, such as a fall. After that, it seems like everything is downhill. Pneumonia pops up, old bouts of shingles reoccur, and so forth. Antibiotics are highly suspect in making the tissue accept infections rather than conquer them. Once accepted, the body no longer fights, and so apparent health is restored. This is known as artificial health.

41

Even vaccinations that only use dead virus to forcibly educate the immune system leave foreign particles in the body, or an incomplete immunilogical response that then leaves some people susceptible to a host of problems and event more dangerous pathogens.

Dr. Moskowitz (Switzerland) hypothesizes that by introducing the vaccine directly into the blood stream, it promotes a deeper, systemic, chronic pathology than a bout of the actual disease itself.

Bypassing the normal mode of entry into the body, the injected vaccination does not stimulate the whole immune system, and virus particles may remain in the tissues. The body's antibodies will now have to be directed to the cell itself which evokes an auto-immune response. By attacking its own genetic material to deal with the immunization (as an episome to the genome of the host cell), the virus particle becomes permanently encoded with the cell's genetic material. These latent viruses, the auto-immune response phenomina, and cancer become pieces of the same puzzle — an incompetent immune system.

What's been presented here may be a little complex for some, a little oversimplified for others, but it is pertinent to our purpose regarding Candidiasis and the immune system.

After vaccination, a person's overall constitution is weakened, but immunity to a specific disease is gained. Rather than strengthening the whole body, the vaccination tricks the body into being non-reactive to one specific disease. The overall effect is an individual one. Some children show little effect. Many have fevers and reactions. Some die. I personally have seen bright-eyed, playful, vital children become dull, clingy, tired, sleepy-headed, and susceptible to colds and respiratory infections after vaccination. Once a homeopathic remedy was given to counter the infectious puncture wound and provide drainage, the former personality and vibrant health returned. Of course this isn't possible for the ones who die — those few and far between statistics based on the erroneous but seemingly necessary philosophy of "sacrifice the few for the sake of the many."

The medical profession thinks it is acceptable for a certain vaccination to be lethal, that is deadly, to a certain percentage of the children taking it — some are .0006% lethal. Let's take one that is only .0001% lethal. That's about the same as lining up 10,000 doctors, giving them each a pistol and saying, "Point this to your head and pull the trigger. Only one pistol is loaded."

Vaccinations have been successful in saving lives and preventing disfigurement, but there is a cost, and more and more people today, including doctors, want to investigate another way — one that builds the whole person's entire immune system.

One last point on vaccinations. The trend in medicine has been to combine vaccinations into one big shot such as DPT or MMR. Never in nature are people exposed to simultaneous plagues. The immune system is programmed to deal with one life-threatening epidemic at a time. By combining major diseases into one shot, the immune system is expected to mount a widely diversified attack. The result may well be confusion, only partial immunity, and susceptibility to even more dangerous forms of pathogenic organisms. Wholistic doctors strive to avoid multiple vaccinations in a single shot for this reason.

A weakened immune system goes hand in hand with candida proliferation, and vice versa, so it's important to be aware of all the factors. Anything that weakens the immune system can allow the opportunistic candida to proliferate. And once weakened, the same substance can inhibit recovery from candidiasis. This is true in some instances of mercury and nickel poisoning from silver amalgam dental fillings, toxic residue from drugs, poor diet, and so forth.

Candidiasis is often referred to as an insidious disease, because of the seriousness of its effects and the fact that it not only weakens the immune system by taxing it, it can actually attack the immune system and destroy immune cells.

Medical science understands a little more about the immune system each year, and giant strides are being made, but there's such a long way to go. The electron microscope is revealing incredible insights into the immune system and advancing our knowledge at a phenomenal pace based on what can be learned by studying dead organisms since the microscope works in a vacuum environment. [What ever happened to the Royal Rife microscope which could view live organisms at a 50,000 magnification that was being used at the Mayo Clinic in the 1940's? Rife found that cancer could be halted by specific electro-magnetic oscillations and his research and microscope "disappeared."]

Looking at the ancient acupuncture charts and oriental healing literature, it is evident that the Chinese also understood a great deal — some four thousand years ago. Of course, their understanding was from an energy perspective rather than a cellular, chemical one. The energy perspective is still being overlooked by medicine today. But the nutritionists are in the enviable position of being able to use knowledge from both systems.

On the subject of acupuncture, it is important to understand that Chinese medicine views candida as a "damp spleen." This is quite fascinating in that candida inhabits the body's damp area (the mucosa) and the mucosa is ruled by the spleen, according to the acupuncture meridian system. In western biology, the spleen is known to be the filter for the lymphatic system and a storage house for lymphocytes (immune system cells), and thus plays a vital role in a person's immune system. It is common knowledge in nutritional circles that western medicine overlooks the importance of the spleen (the often-exhibited "if we don't know what it does, cut it out" mentality) and that current research is showing the spleen to be a critically important, but little understood organ.

The thymus gland (located in the middle of the chest) is a fairly recent discovery for today's medicine. Now, with the immune system under attack from so many enemies (natural enemies, such as bacteria, parasites, and viruses, and human-made enemies like pesticides, amalgam dental fillings, toxic drugs, environmental pollution, radiation, etc.), a great deal of attention is being paid to it.

Briefly, cells that function as our mobile immune system are derived from two areas — the bone marrow (macrophages, neutrophyls, macrophasias, basophils, eosinophils), and the lymph nodes/spleen system (lymphocytes). Each type of cell has a specific function, just like different components of an army have specific, yet synergistic functions — scouting, communicating, attacking, cleaning up, and so forth.

A third and most critical aspect of the immune system is the inherent cellular immunity. Each individual cell has a defense system. This could be likened to your home security system of dead bolts, strong doors, lights, shotgun over the fireplace, etc. The other mobile immune cells could be likened to the police, state militia, national guard, armed forces, and state department all providing for the common defense. Cellular immunity is dependent upon nutrition (protein, vitamins C, A, B-group, organic minerals) and electrical charge (bio-electrical properties). An emphasis must be placed on usable amino acids (protein) for it's vital role in the strengthening of the cell and it's immunity. Also, the collagen, which holds the cells together, is composed of a triple helix molecule of glycine, proline, and hydroxyproline — another protein-dependent part of our natural immunity.

Now somewhere in the annals of medical history, doctors decided that the thymus gland was a vestigial organ — one that is most active in protecting the body after the colostrum (first mother's milk) stops flowing, around the third day, through about age 14, at which time it shrinks, having accomplished most of its immunity work. This is true, but now the findings are that the thymus plays a critical role in adult immunity as well.

Similar thinking enshrouds the appendix, the tonsils, and adenoids. Medicine thinks either 1) that God made useless and troublesome parts of the body or, 2) that Nature/evolution has progressed our species beyond the need for these body parts. The result of this thinking is the same — "cut them out." Let's not be so hasty to write off our body parts.

Nutritionists have known for some time now that the appendix provides a lubricant for the colon and that the tonsils are an early warning system for detecting bacteria proliferation in the oral/sinus cavities. The appendix, tonsils, and adenoids are just now being recognized as parts of the immune system — reservoirs for lymphatic cells. Nutritionists also know from Chinese acupuncture that the thymus is of major importance to the adult body. Naturopathic philosophy has it that the blueprint for the body is perfect (or pretty close to perfect), that the various parts should stay intact, and that the causes of their congestion (impaired function) should be treated, not just the symptoms suppressed or cut out.

Candidiasis affects the immune system in several ways:

1. Controlling yeast is one of the first immune battles the newborn infant fights. Antibodies are formed based on the immu-

nologic response of the thymus-derived cells and B-lymphocytes. From birth, the immune system has a job keeping yeast under control. An equilibrium is established and maintained throughout life until something unbalances it.

2. Yeast/fungus proliferation can stress the immune system beyond its ability to function properly. The continual exposure causes a situation called "tolerance induction," which means the immune system gets used to the candida in the blood and tissues and no longer fights wholeheartedly. It gets tired. This allows the yeast/fungus to colonize throughout the body. In this state the immune system is paralyzed and unable to respond adequately to any call for help.

3. In its fungal form, candida can overcome the cellular immune system (the most basic and most important part of the immune system) and then invade and destroy tissue.

4. Yeast/fungus can attack and alter the T-cells (thymus-derived or thymus-activated white blood cells including T-helpers and T-suppressors). In AIDS, the ratio between T-helpers (fighters) and T-suppressors (peacemakers) becomes unbalanced so there are too many T-suppressors, meaning the immune system weakens itself and inhibits its own immune response. Toxins released from candida/fungus can alter the T-cells and confuse the immune system's response. Medical research found that candida can suppress natural killer cells (soldiers of the immune system) and form new auto-immune complexes. The toxins (antigens) from candida can combine with the immune system's antibodies, causing inflammatory and tissue-destroying action.

5. Candida's by-products are very toxic. They poison the system with hundreds of toxic chemicals, such as acetaldehyde, and the immune system and liver must labor to control the level of toxins. If the level becomes too high, infection of the central nervous system can occur.

Research is also looking for a virus-antigen as a participant in this destructive pattern. For the last five years, our research has found that virus is involved with candidiasis (perhaps the virus that causes Epstein- Barr), and thus we include antiviral factors in people's nutritional approaches to overcoming candida.

46

The seriousness of this type of disease cannot be emphasized enough. Destruction and distortion of the immune system can only lead to misery and death.

Candidiasis is the forerunner of immune-deficient diseases such as AIDS and others yet to come. There is some speculation that the 50,000 genetic experimental labs around the world may be releasing new, virulent strains of micro-organisms into the biosphere. A great deal of research continues as the world's superpowers apply biology to warfare.

If the disease pattern that we see with AIDS and candida continues, the only ones who'll survive are those with strong immune systems. So let's learn what weakens or strengthens our immune systems so we can meet these challenges.

It is fundamentally and critically important to conquer candidiasis NOW and work nutritionally to strengthen the immune system to have a healthy life.

People should pay attention to the new nutritional findings regarding the immune system. For instance, research on coenzyme Q-10 shows that this relative of vitamin K can improve cellular energy (immunity) and it helps the rate at which phagocytes (white blood cells) clear foreign matter from the body.

The herb echinacea stimulates the immune system temporarily (until homeostasis renders it ineffective in about 10-14 days) and can be used in short cycles to improve the body's immune response.

Homeopathic potentizations of the mineral silica (silicea) prove to increase macrophage activity.

Oxygen increases lymphocyte viability so the mineral germanium, as well as stabilized oxygen (not hydrogen peroxide), are promising immune assistants.

Sensitivities To Aldehydes

People with candidiasis often complain of sensitivities to perfumes, odors, and fragrances. Such people are often labeled "environmental sensitives" and may need to go to such extremes as moving to the country, wearing gas masks, removing carpets from their homes, wearing only cotton clothing, and eating only specific foods.

These supersensitive people often lack the nutrients used in the metabolic processing of aldehydes (chemical fragrances), such as niacin, niacinamide, riboflavin, molybdenum, and iron.

Aldehydes are often processed in the body with the essential amino acid threonine, which makes the toxic chemical, acetaldehyde, which in turn is processed into acetic acid and on into acetyl coenzyme A. An enzyme known as aldehyde oxidase is specifically dedicated to this process.

It is interesting to note that alcohol is processed by a similar method. The abundance of the toxic acetaldehyde damages the tissues far more than the alcohol.

Acetaldehyde is a by-product of the carbohydrates that are fermented by yeast. In the body, fermentations cause poisons and cancer, and in the case of candida, the acetaldehydes produced by its metabolic processes can cause environmental sensitivities.

More than any other nutrient, the trace mineral molybdenum helps support the neutralization of acetaldehydes. It also helps neutralize sulfites used as food preservatives. The recommended doseage is 100-300 mcg. per day, along with sea-based, broad spectrum mineral supplementation. Foods which, if properly grown, contain molybdenum include buckwheat, lima beans, liver, barley, oats, lentils, and sunflower seeds.

THE CAUSES OF AND CONTRIBUTORS TO CANDIDIASIS

According to Dr. Orion Truss, author of *The Hidden Diagnosis* and pioneer in the treatment of candidiasis, the primary causes of this disease are antibiotics, birth control pills, and immune-suppressive drugs. There are just a few things that cause candidiasis and a host of things that contribute to it. The primary causes are antibiotics, birth control pills, steroids/cortisone, failure to breast-feed, and, perhaps, the persistent use of soap on the skin. The other topics discussed here are important considerations, but secondary contributors rather than causes.

There is a great deal of confusion about what causes candidiasis and what contributes to it. "Causes" are serious considerations, "contributors" are serious aggravators.

Causes of Candidiasis Overview

Alkaline soaps (subcutaneous candida)

Antibiotics (in food and medicine)

Birth control pills (steroids)

High blood sugar (diabetes)

Immune deficiency (inherited or acquired)

Failure to breast-feed

Steroids (anti-inflammatory) cortisone

Contributors of Candidiasis Overview
(weakens the immune system)

Addictive substances (caffeine, alcohol, sugar)

Chlorine/fluoride in tap water

Chronic Allergic Reactions

Detrimental (non-loving) attitudes

High carbohydrate diet

Improper colonics (using chlorinated water)

Liver function, impaired

Musty, moldy climate/environment

Silver amalgam dental fillings

Stress, excessive

Subclinical infections (herpes, Epstein-Barr)

Toxins (excessive) in the system

Vaccinations

In some ways, the current candida pandemic is due to the cumulative effect of all the items listed above. So let's begin with the now-abandoned movement sponsored by the American Medical Association to stop mothers from breast-feeding their babies and find out why the 1950's babies are prone to 1980's candida.

The Failure to Breast-feed and the Importance of Colostrum (Cause)

Back in the 1940s and 50s, medical journals advocated the use of formulas instead of mother's milk as the ideal food for infants. Many news articles and doctors' recommendations discouraged breast feeding in favor of human-designed formulas based on cow's milk instead of human milk. Some suspect that there may have been connections between these recommendations and the dairy industry via political lobbies, and the usual debased monetary motivations. [You'll note that today there is a push to sell cow's milk to the public due to overproduction. Many nutritionists take a strong stand against milk as a beneficial food, as it's found in stores today — pasteurized and homogenized. It certainly does NOT provide usable calcium. (See: *The Pro-Vita! Plan*)

The companies that made baby formula sent millions of samples to doctors to give to new mothers to relieve them from the "pain and inconvenience" of breast feeding.

I know it's hard to believe from the perspective of the 1980s that the public could ever be so gullible as to believe breast feeding was inferior to a commercial formula. It's hard to believe the medical profession could be so arrogant as to propose that it knows better than Nature how to feed an infant.

But this no-breast feeding movement came at a time when it seemed medicine could conquer all illness and provide long and healthy lives. And the public was chasing the idea of science providing convenience in the form of appliances and a higher standard of living. Now we see quite a different story, as the medical labor union (A.M.A) is struggling to hold people in its thrall, discriminating against nutritionally-oriented doctors, searching to provide drug-oriented answers for the many problems it created.

The myth is shattering, and candidiasis is making the public aware that a change is needed.

When an infant first nurses, it receives a substance known as colostrum, which helps establish the intestinal flora, as well as immune factors. Colostrum is high in proteins, antibodies, and contains a trace of hydrogen peroxide. During this time, the infant's stomach acids are not as strong as they'll be in a few days, so the colostrum bacteria easily passes into the G.I. tract where they hybridize, stick, and form a healthy environment. This helps seed the small and large intestine with beneficial bacteria. After a few nursings, milk production starts and the infant's stomach acids develop an incredibly strong digesting medium that makes milk assimilable.

Note: calcium is assimilable only in an acid environment. Milk neutralizes acid, so to benefit from calcium in milk, infants must have very strong acid, and they do. After weaning, the stomach acids reduce to a higher pH (less acidic). This is one reason that milk is not such a good source of calcium for adults, contrary to what the TV advertisements tell us. Also, this is why the popular product Tums, an antacid designed to neutralize stomach acid, cannot provide usable calcium as the TV advertisements claim.

One more point on antacids. They are considered non-systemic since they do not alter blood bicarbonate levels, but they do alter urine pH, making it more alkaline. Cystitis, urinary tract yeast infections, and bladder infections occur in an alkaline environment and could well result from antacid use. Frequent need to use antacids is often indicative of candidiasis in the stomach.

It's important to note that colostrum contains the antibodies that help establish the infant's immunity to many diseases. Also it is sticky, which means it adheres to the intestinal walls, unlike the cultures (acidophilus, lactobacillus, bifidus, bulgaricus, thermophilus) people use to try to replace the bacteria lost to antibiotics.

THE INTESTINAL CULTURE FORMED AT BIRTH FROM THE FIRST NURSINGS OF COLOSTRUM BECOMES THE PERSON'S OWN, UNIQUE CULTURE. IT ADAPTS TO THE INFANT'S BODY AND BECOMES A PART OF ITS ECOLOGICAL SYSTEM. This is important to understand, as the re-seeding of the G.I. tract is quite difficult. Taking cultures can help a little, but they are not the exact, right culture for a person's individual system. Many acidophilus cultures sold are not normally found in human beings.

So if your mother did not breast-feed you (due to inability or upon recommendation by a doctor), you did not have your G.I. tract properly seeded with beneficial bacteria. This means you are more susceptible to candida proliferation than people who have well-established, beneficial intestinal flora. Also, without colostrum, the immune system was established without all the cards in the deck. This may have given you a predisposition to sensitivities, asthma, allergies, hayfever, and so forth. And as we now know, the immune system helps prevent candidiasis and is adversely affected by it's proliferation. Not breast-feeding causes double jeopardy.

Antibiotics (Cause)

In societies of medical orientation, people take tetracyclines and other antibiotics for ear infections, acne, colds, and infections of the respiratory, urinary, and vaginal areas. Many dentists wield antibiotics for precautionary purposes even when no infection is present. Since the intestinal culture is so important for our resistance to disease, our ability to absorb and synthesize nutrients, and our ultimate health, what happens when broad-spectrum antibiotics kill off the beneficial bacteria? Once the lifetime supply of colostrum-based bacteria is killed, IT'S GONE. And most people's diets and food combining patterns support the growth of putrefactive bacteria. It all adds up to dysbiosis of the G.I. tract.

To make matters even worse where antibiotics are concerned, candida thrives on tetracyclines as a food source! Many antibiotics not only kill the beneficial bacteria that keep the yeast in check, they feed the yeast/fungus, causing proliferation.

Furthermore, there is new evidence that antibiotics actually damage the cellular immunity, making the cells easier to penetrate and thus more susceptible to future infections. Antibiotics fed to poultry push so much salmonella and botulism (food poisoning) organisms into the birds' tissues that unless poultry is first given a Chlorox bath (see The Pro-Vita *Plan*)and cooked very well, food poisoning and salmonella can occur as these organisms are increasingly inherent in the meat.

Attempts are being made to re-seed colostrum bacteria in the G.I. tract, but so far have been unsuccessful. Adults cannot accomplish this by taking colostrum, because the stomach acid kills it

Rectal implants will not reach the small intestine, and time-release properties haven't worked yet either, as the proper strains for an individual are somewhat unique — a hybrid of more than one kind of culture that has its birth shortly after the breast-feeding infant's birth. Time released cultures are introduced to a hostile environment rather than the pristine environment of a newborn.

But nutritional labs have been working on this. They will have to find some kind of sticky, viable bacteria culture that can be delivered in a time release form to get it past the stomach acids and duodenal alkali and into the small intestine. Research efforts have centered around attempts to crossbreed colostrum bacteria with raw sauerkraut (acid-resilient) bacteria to form a sticky, beneficial culture with which to re-seed the G.I. tract. As of this writing, results have been elusive, and such a formula is not yet available. The latest word is that it may be more practical to take the two cultures separately and let them work it out in the G.I. tract on their own. This has given rise to the therapy of taking acidophilus in the evening and bifidus first thing in the morning.

As of 1989, this is still the most viable approach to improving the intestinal culture. Supplements which provide several culures in a single capsule are not as successful perhaps because they are providing competetive cultures at the same time, or perhaps because they do not refrigerate their cultures.

People who use antibiotics have weakened intestinal cultures and have tendencies toward candida proliferation. There's still the immune system to keep it in check, but candida is relentless. The degree of candidiasis infection is based upon how much a person's immune system can handle and what they do to support it or tax their system. Birth control pills, improper diet, nutritional deficiencies, exposure to pesticides (agriculturally and on foods in supermarkets), cortisone-type drugs, subclinical infections (herpes, Epstein-Barr, vaccinations), miasmic (constitutionally-inherited) weaknesses, silver amalgam dental fillings (they leak mercury and cause electrical current), radiation, chemotherapy, and addictive substances (tobacco, alcohol, caffeine, sugar), all tax and weaken the immune system.

One other consideration is the chlorine and flouride added to tap water and its effect on the G.I. tract. Nutritionists have long known these chemicals rob vitamin E from the body, as well as contribute to altered bacteria cultures. Inorganic flourides, such as the kind used in many city waters and toothpastes, are suspect in candidiasis. It's difficult to get the research out, since many dentists promote flouride in public drinking water as well as in toothpastes. Since the flouride controversies of the early 1970s, this issue has been smouldering and will probably resurface in a few years. It's an old argument based on public freedom and the difference between "organic" flouride from plants and "inorganic" flouride from chemicals.

For a growing number of people it's a moot point as they employ water purification equipment (reverse osmosis and various other filters) in their homes and offices, as far as drinking water goes, but people have yet to realize the toxic effects of bathing in polluted water.

How recent are the reports linking candidiasis and broad-spectrum antibiotics? As early as 1951 a report came out regarding the antibiotic Aureomycin . Researchers McVay and Sprunt tested 186 patients, all initially free of candida proliferation. After using the antibiotic, 117 subjects developed candidiasis. Such information went unheeded or it was explained away by saying that candida

54

was only behaving as an opportunistic organism, and the body would soon bring it under control when all infection was cleared up. Now there are reports that show candidiasis is a common factor in AIDS. So far, these reports are going unheeded by most doctors. Fortunately people are addressing the problem of candida, thanks to an increasing nutritional awareness and to a few nutritional pioneers.

Aureomycin hit the market in 1947. If you go back through the medical journals of 1948 through 1960, you'll find numerous reports and concerns about major increases in vaginal and intestinal yeast infections. Following the same correlation, candidiasis became pandemic after the introduction of the anti-fertility, birth control pill.

Now, in the late 1980s, new antibiotics are being used that are much more specific. Rather than being broad-spectrum, they target specific microorganisms. It is thought that these drugs do not disturb the intestinal flora as much because they are specific only to a particular bacteria. But they still are responsible for breeding new, more resistant strains, as they do not work with the body's natural laws of cure.

It remains to be seen what side effects these drugs will have, but they do seem to be vastly improved over the broad-spectrum drugs. One of these antibiotics, nystatin, is a specific against candida and forms the cornerstone of the medical approach to killing candida in the G.I. tract and vaginal areas. More on this in the "Treatment" section.

People try to re-seed the G.I. tract with beneficial cultures in supplement form and, while there is some good accomplished by this, some researchers claim much of the supplemental bacteria are killed in the stomach IF they were viable to begin with after sitting on a store's shelf for who knows how long. Not being a sticky bacteria, supplemental cultures pass out with the feces, and thus they must be perpetually administered, usually for years, in hopes the body will accept them as a resident culture.

Even so, taking beneficial cultures is important as we'll see in the chapter on treatment. This is particularly important for people who 1) were not breast-fed, 2) have taken antibiotics or birth control pills, and 3) have eaten a lot of meat, such as commercial beef, pork, chicken, and turkey, treated with antibiotics. It's also important for people who have suppressed their immune systems with energy-addictive substances (coffee, sugar, tobacco, marijuana, chocolate, and others). [See *The Next Step To Greater Energy* (Tips)]

Such addictive substances stimulate the adrenal glands to produce adrenalin and other hormones that suppress the thymus gland, which is the heart of the immune system. With a weakened immune system, invasive fungus is better able to colonize and cause candidiasis.

While on the subject of the adrenal glands, let's take a brief look at the body's biochemistry. The mineral copper is a natural fungicide. It is often used in swimming pools to control molds and algae. The body's copper needs to be "organic" and available, as it is an oxygenator. When the adrenal glands are weak, copper is stored in certain tissue and becomes unavailable, or it may simply become deficient. In either case, this anti-fungal oxygen-carrying mineral is not available to perform its functions. To truly overcome candidiasis and have it not return, the endocrine glands must be nourished and stabilized at a good level of performance.

Many people wonder whether the antibiotics in animal feed, as well as those injected into these animals, contribute to candidiasis. The answer is an emphatic YES. Few people realize that around 42% of all the antibiotics produced in the United States go into animal feed. This massive dose is passed on to you if you eat commercial meat, eggs, cheeses, milk, and ice cream. Perhaps it's time to investigate chemical-free meats and reduce the amount eaten. Consumers should control the market. More requests for chemical-free produce can result in more being available.

In March, 1987, the popular American TV show "60 Minutes" ran a feature on the poultry industry and the high levels of toxic salmonella bacteria (food poisoning) found in the meat. The program emphasized sanitation, processing, and cover-ups.

Although this is an important part of the picture it is by no means the whole of it.

If we look at this from the perspective that holds that the antibiotics push disease deeper into the cells and tissues, then the rampant salmonella infestation in poultry could well be due to the antibiotics administered in the birds' feed.

This means the salmonella could well be dormant or suppressed into the tissues, to become active again after the chicken is slaughtered.

It is important to cook chicken throughly to destroy the salmonella. Also, the skin is quite toxic, as the fats become rancid and carcinogenic when cooked. The rules here are: If you eat chicken, it should be organically raised, you should not use the skin, and you should cook it thoroughly. The already mentioned Chlorox or hydrogen peroxide bath is essential prior to cooking as explained in the book "The Pro-Vita Plan".

We should ask, "why do chickens need antibiotics in the first place?" Nature provides the chicken with a well-functioning immune system capable of controlling bacteria. It is the unnatural environment the commercial chicken is raised in that causes great imbalances. Chickens are stacked in cages and never touch the ground or interact with each other. They are exposed to artificial light (to alter the day-night rhythms) to make them lay more eggs. They are fed growth steroids, which cause bacteria proliferation, and so they must be fed antibiotics to control the bacteria.

Similar conditions exist with commercial beef and pork. No wonder people suffer a decline in health when they overeat the flesh of such neurotic and artificially raised animals. Also, it's interesting to reflect on the similarities between food-animal stresses (overpopulation, artificial diet, inoculations, etc.) to 20th Century human stresses.

Antibiotic Overview

Antibiotics:

• Create new, more virulent, more resistant strains of bacteria
• Feed candida-fungus
• Force the body to accept disease deep in the tissue
• Contribute to chronic-degenerative disease
• Weaken cellular immunity and the immune system
• Destroy the beneficial bacteria in the G.I. tract and vagina
• Deplete nutrients (B vitamins)
• Cause vaginal infections
• Cause Candidiasis
• Break the natural immune cycle wherebythe body learns how to recognize and control pathogens.

What is needed now is a new understanding of how we treat the body. This is not a call to banish antibiotics; only a call for a new perspective on when to use such a weapon.

One part of the creed of the naturopath is "Do No Harm." And fortunately there is little need to ever require an antibiotic.

A strong immune system is the first step to avoiding the need for antibiotics.

Should an infection take hold, there are plenty of natural therapies to help the body correct it such as homeopathic remedies, anti-infective herbs, and cleansing diets. And these natural remedies work exceedingly well! Oftentimes they work as quickly as antibiotics (particularly for those following a healthful lifestyle) and the body emerges stronger and wiser than before.

Proper natural care would mean perhaps only one out of ten million people would ever require an antibiotic to avoid the effects of a life-threatening disease.

So step one - the strong immune system - is the place to start since our immune systems are being compromised daily due to the environment and stress.

Strengthen your immune system and use natural remedies, live a healthful lifestyle, and you may never need an antibiotic.

This isn't good news for the pharmaceutical industry, or for the doctors who prefer to treat every symptom with an antibiotic rather than treat the person as an individual, but this is good news for you and your quality of life.

Birth Control Pills/Steroids (Cause)

As already mentioned, a chronological scan of medical journals shows that concern about Candidiasis began shortly after the introduction of antibiotics. A quantum leap in concern occurred after the introduction of the anti-fertility (birth control) pill.

Someday history may attribute to the birth control pill the distinction of being the greatest cause of Candidiasis — even more so than antibiotics.

Birth control pills (estrogen/progesterone) and steroids (cortisone) are immune-suppressive drugs. We already know that when

58

the immune system is compromised, opportunistic yeast can become fungal-invasive and cause problems.

Perhaps one reason women are more affected by candidiasis than men is that their natural progesterone levels swing high in the luteal phase of menstruation. Another reason is that the vaginal area provides an additional, "external" environment suitable (warm, moist) for yeast to colonize.

Birth control pills should be discontinued. Notify your doctor. The new cervical cap provides effective contraception without side effects.

Candidiasis can cause an altered immune system and women can become allergic to their own hormones (estrogen and progesterone) since candida has receptor sites for these hormones. Such an allergy may require homeopathic neutralization during the anticandida program.

Drugs that weaken the immune system and provide an environment favorable to candida are in no way safe, even though the so-called "studies" by the pharmaceutical manufacturers tell us birth control pills are safe, or as the latest hype tells us - can even help prevent cancer.

High Carbohydrate Diet (Contributor)

Americans are eating more carbohydrates than ever before. Complex carbohydrates include starches (potatoes, rice, whole grain breads, oat meal, grains, beans cooked at the boiling point, pasta, and so forth). Highly refined carbohydrates include cakes, white bread, pies, potato chips, desserts, candy, sodas, and most of the typical junk foods. Stu Wheelwright tells people, "You're not a dough boy. Your body is built on protein and water with a little carbohydrate in transit for energy."

Complex carbohydrates provide a good fuel for the body when they are in a proper matrix of amino acids, but they do not build the immune system. Read the *Pro-Vita! Diet* for in depth dietary research.

High carbohydrate diets mean there's an abundance of sugars to support yeast proliferation. Diabetics inevitably have difficulty with candida because their blood sugar levels are high.

In addition to high carbohydrate intake, people also eat sugars, which further adds to the yeast-support environment.

An overly high carbohydrate diet means low cellular protein, low immunity, weakened connective tissue, and lowered bio-energy. This is a major problem for vegetarians who rely on carbohydrate combinations (beans and rice) to try to get their protein. The cellular matrix (the energy blueprint) changes to a "make-do" instead of a "make it right" pattern, which results in the gradual decline of energy. Most sugar/carbohydrate cravings are really a signal that proteins are either lacking in the diet or are not being broken down to nucleo-proteins so they can be used by the cells. Vegetarians must use soaked seed combinations along with tofu and perhaps some fish occasionally to maintain protein integrity. This is based on clinical experience — not on conjecture.

This does not mean that people need a high protein diet (which can lead to other problems). It means proteins must be used properly. This is discussed in *The Pro-Vita! Plan*.

Diets high in refined carbohydrates (typical of junk food diets) are also low in fiber, so another anti-candida factor is missing. The beneficial bacteria prefer higher fiber levels than most people get in their diets. The harmful bacteria prefer the concentrated sugars, the putrefactive meats, and improperly combined foods, which will ferment because proper digestion cannot take place.

Toxins In The Tissues (Contributor)

Toxins such as agricultural pesticides, environmental pollutants (auto exhaust, lead, tobacco and marijuana smoke, hair spray, industrial wastes), fermentations of protein in the bowel, heavy metals (mercury from dental fillings, aluminum from antiperspirants, cadmium from paint, tobacco, marijuana, etc.), medicinal drugs, and so forth, can be stored in body tissues when the liver is sluggish or the kidneys stressed. Toxic areas foster the colonization of yeast/fungus. [Remember the wolf and the reindeer? Candida is attracted to the weakened areas.]

To detoxify the body according to its natural pathways, read *Your Liver ... Your Lifeline* (Tips. 1993).

Musty, Moldy Climate/Environment (Contributor)

Damp, moldy environments contribute to Candidiasis by encouraging airborne yeasts and molds. Regarding the mold issue, this means that living in dry, mountain air is better for candida patients than is living on a houseboat in the bayous.

People with Candidiasis should avoid musty basements and moldy leaves, and so forth, until their immune systems are strong enough to handle such exposures.

Silver-Amalgam Dental Fillings (Contributor)

In spite of strenuous efforts on the part of the American Dental Association to suppress information regarding the hazards and potential hazards of silver-amalgam dental fillings, word is finally out to the public, thanks to the efforts of Drs. Hal Huggins and Sam Ziff, who have published popular books on this subject.

There are two ways amalgam fillings can hurt the immune system — one is by releasing toxic metals (mercury and nickel primarily) into the body. The other is by generating enough galvanic current to disrupt the nerve and meridian energy flow, which travels through the thymus gland.

The galvanic current causes the release of toxic metals. If the liver is not functioning well enough (few peoples' are today) to chelate toxins and detoxify the body, the toxic metals will be stored in the brain, liver, kidney, adipose tissues, as well as in the lymphatic fluid.

Whether or not fillings are a problem depends on the individual circumstances — what metals are in the amalgam and for instance, the position of the fillings, how pitted the surface of the fillings are, how acid the diet is, and how strong the liver and lymphatic functions are, to name a few.

But there is no doubt that the fillings disrupt the body's bio-energetic system and contribute to the toxic load on the immune system.

Teeth are actually quite porous and the filling materials pass through them into the body.

In clinical testing with electro-acupuncture equipment designed for this purpose, we've measured high galvanic current in small, single fillings and, suprisingly, found very little in some people with numerous fillings. As for determining the amount of toxic metals in the system, a hair analysis by a reliable lab can provide insights into tissue levels. We used to advise that before removing and replacing silver-amalgam fillings, it is advisable to first evaluate how high a priority it is. Now with several more years of research to base opinions on, the issue is of even greater importance. It's really best to not have silver amalgum dental fillings.

An interesting note, the metallic silver has an anti-gram-positive bacterial, anti-streptococcus-mutants effect, which can protect the tooth from decay under the filling. Perhaps the ideal filling would be a composite, like Occlusin with a touch of pure silver and gold (also an antibiotic in miniscule amounts for gram-negative bacteria).

The reason people fail to understand how a little bitty dental filling can ruin their health is they don't understand the electrical or bio-energetic properties of the body. Even the high-speed dental drill can cause a disruptive energy flow into the delicate meridian energy system.

Once fillings are removed, the body can detoxify itself of mercury — often causing reactions. This usually occurs in 21-day cycles. Enzymated vitamin C, such as sago palm vitamin C in a base of clove and cinnamon, can help ease mercury deposits from the tissues and chelate them, usually with the amino acid glutamine, for export out of the body. Homeopathics also work well for releasing the heavy metals. Kidney support available from your health professinal such as Systemic Formulas' K (Kidney), ACX (Vitamin Detox), and CTV (Therapeutic Vitamin C with thymol iodide) are particularly useful and often recommended during metal-detoxification programs.

Improperly Applied Colonic Irrigations (Contributor)

Once while traveling with Wheelwright, he consulted with 45 people in west Texas who had been on numerous and frequent colonic irrigations (a therapy that involves washing out the colon with water). He pointed out these people were amazingly free of chronic, degenerative diseases, such as arthritis and cancer. Most, however, were rampant with candida in the gastrointestinal (G.I.) tract.

We inspected the colonic equipment and found it was hooked up to the town's tap water. The chlorine and alkaline pH of the water interfered with the beneficial bacteria and, although it cleansed the bowel of poisonous debris, it contributed to an unhealthy bacteria environment.

Colonics are a beneficial therapy, a health science of their own, but they must be properly applied. The water should be free of chlorine and slightly acidic (pH 6.85-6.90). It is a good idea to implant chlorophyll or bifidus at the end to promote the beneficial bacteria's repopulation.

Some other suggestions about colonics include, implanting lactobacillus cultures and making the water slightly saline (1 tsp. sea salt per gallon). This will help reduce the possibility of absorbing toxins, as the salt water will have a slight hydrogogue effect and pull body water into the colon for expulsion. Since the salt water is close to the specific gravity of the blood, it will not be absorbed by osmosis into the body. Some colonic therapists add fresh oxygen to the water to kill anaerobic bacteria and parasites. Some use a touch of hydroxylquinalin sulfate acid (from grapefruit rind and seed) to reinstate the natural acid mantle and inhibit fungal growth.

LEVELS OF CANDIDIASIS

Infection with Candida progresses through several levels. The first level involves the acceptance of yeast by the infant's body shortly after birth, when the immune system sets up its controls. This is a moot level, or level zero, since we all live in a sea of yeast.

There is no official line of demarcation between levels of Candidasis involvement, so they are only general categories that show how much the yeast/fungus is stressing the body and to what degree the system is affected.

Candidiasis Level One. Infections in the G.I. and genitourinary tracts marked by any number of symptoms including diarrhea, constipation, bloating, heartburn, gas, indigestion, white coating on tongue, sorethroats, cystitis, anal itching, vaginitis, malabsorption of nutrients, yeast infections, weight gain, and genital rashes.

Candidiasis Level Two. Infections and toxins pass into the bloodstream and cause immune system breakdown and allergies to foods and environment. When this occurs, the body can react with hives, headaches, rashes, acne, asthma, hay fever, ear infections, weight gain, bronchitis, colds, and fatigue.

Candidiasis Level Three. Central nervous system dysfunction and deterioration occurs because of excessive toxins in the bloodstream — some of which interfere with nerve synapse transmissions. Symptoms include memory loss or lapses, headaches, depression, PMS, irritability, belligerence, lack of concentration, fatigue, lack of motivation, poor self- image, confusion, and being spacey.

Candidiasis Level Four. Endocrine gland and organ breakdown occurs. As the nerve impulses fail, communication between the many parts of the body breaks down. Endocrine gland responses become weak. The thyroid and adrenal glands (energy glands) become underactive. The hypothalmus miscommunicates. Also, the gonads (ovaries, testes) become stressed, causing further glandular imbalance. Fungus invades these weakened tissues causing physical damage to the tissue. Parts of the body are literally eaten alive. Symptoms include hypothyroidism, adrenal burnout, severe fatigue, severe abdominal pain, PMS, menstrual irregularities (endometriosis, amenorrhea, dysmenorrhea), infertility, lack of breast development, and low liver function. At this level, all therapies have a tendency to aggravate the condition, making it difficult to get started on a program.

DIAGNOSING CANDIDIASIS

Candidiasis has been named the "missing diagnosis" by Dr. Orion Truss because of the difficulty in pinpointing it. Its symptoms are so varied that medical science did not suspect that they could come from the same source. An opportunistic organism, candida increases when the immune system is weak or when it is stressed by fighting off some other problem.

A great debt is owed to Dr. Orion Truss for showing how candidiasis can be the one cause of so many problems. Weakened immunity allows the candidiasis to flourish.

As people became plagued with candidiasis, they were often told by their doctors that their symptoms of depression, fatigue, and light-headedness were "all in their heads." Many were referred to psychotherapists and allergists, or they simply went home confused, without knowing what to do.

Imagine how a fourteen-year-old girl would feel about being told by her doctor that her lack of ability to concentrate, her poor performance in school, her severe depressions, and her fatigue were all imaginary, that she should go see a psychiatrist who'd discuss feelings and prescribe antidepressants (mind-altering drugs). If only a doctor would say, "Something's obviously affecting you, but I do not have the expertise or diagnostic equipment to find out what it is. I recommend you work with a nutritionist who will help support your whole body systemically, so it can repair itself." [We nutritionists have such dreams.]

When candida proliferation was finally noticed, and anti-candida drugs (nystatin) administered, patients improved and their symptoms vanished for a period of time. This started showing the connection between yeast-fungus and a host of illnesses.

Since candidiasis was difficult to diagnose, the standard procedure for finding it was to give patients nystatin and see if they got better. If they did, then the condition was diagnosed as candidiasis.

Today there are quite a few tests for candidiasis — some accurate, some so-so, and some consistently inaccurate.

To diagnose candida, you should first have a suspicion that it might be the problem. Two questionnaires are provided in the next section that will prove helpful to see if there is reason to be suspicious.

Certain people are more likely to have candidiasis. It affects women more than men, and women with multiple pregnancies have an even higher possibility. People with a history of antibiotic use, birth control pills use, cortisone (steroids), and recreational drug use all have greater likelihood of candida being a factor in their health. Also, diabetes mellitus, other prolonged illnesses, radiation, and chemotherapy treatments all predispose people to candidiasis. Note: For some reason people who've had chemotherapy or radiation treatments do not respond well to nystatin. Often other anti-fungal drugs are prescribed.

People with high intakes of sweets, caffeine, fried foods, and alcohol (all the things usually classified as junk foods that lack nutrition and stress the body) provide the proper environment for candida growth. These items are known to be highly stressful — they tax the body both chemically and energetically.

There are many tests to see if a person should suspect that they might have candidiasis. Symptoms that cannot be explained have led many people to seek treatment for candidiasis. One thing to keep in mind is that there are many varieties of candida, and hundreds more varieties of fungus, that may all cause similar symptoms. In clinical practice we know that when a person does not respond well to candida remedies, oftentimes a therapy for other kinds of fungus or parasites will bring the desired results.

Ways of diagnosing candidiasis include taking cultures from anywhere along the G.I. tract (mouth, nose, throat, rectum), from skin lesions, from the genital area, and so forth. Blood or feces are cultured depending on the test the health professional orders.

There is much doubt about the reliability of cultures because, as we've pointed out, yeast is everywhere. And since yeast is a normal inhabitant of the G.I. tract, it is possible to culture it even though it is not causing a problem. Should a culture not show candida, then the evidence is fairly good that the person is not infected at the area the culture was taken from, but this is not conclusive for other areas.

Also, blood lab tests and stool specimen tests offer a low degree of accuracy in locating the symbiotic parasites, entamoeba and giardia. The reason is that these parasites are often embedded in the intestinal mucosa. The only chance for an accurate medical test for entamoeba and giardia is obtained by swabbing the rectal mucosa. This is done with an anoscope and amounts to a superficial biopsy. After centrifuging, a trained lab specimen examiner must identify the forms of giardia.

The blood test (double immunodiffusion) for candida antibodies is more conclusive. If higher than normal levels of precipitins (antibodies) are detected, it can be assumed that the immune system is fighting candida infection at the time. This test also shows the effectiveness of a candida program, because when the battle is over, precipitins will not show in the blood. So people do have a way to test whether and when their nutrition or drug therapy has succeeded.

Blood Tests

Some labs offer a screening assay for the IgG, IgM, and IgA factors specific to candida, which are useful in determining acute and chronic problems with the disease.

Some labs conduct an assay of the amino acids in the blood sample and can predict with a high degree of accuracy whether or not candidiasis is a problem.

As a quick screening, a lab technician who analyzes blood under a microscope can determine if fungus is present by treating a few drops of blood with potassium hydroxide, which lets fungal elements be seen. These can be examined for the familiar cell-invasive fungi.

Dark-field Microscopy

One particularly interesting blood screening technique employs a dark-field microscope, which can transfer the microscopic image to a TV screen so the patient can be shown the candida fungus and a photo can be taken. Then, after therapy, this process can be repeated for comparison, and the patient can see the results. This type of test can be conducted in a progressive nutrition clinic and does not involve delays, high costs, or traumatic blood-drawings. It's relatively easy, practically painless, and quite fascinating. Some thirty other conditions can also be viewed, such as iron deficiency, vitamin E deficiency, immune system deficiencies, high triglycerides, liver congestion, toxic metals, and even suspected virus involvement as seen in lymphocytes.

When dark-field microscopy first announced that candida/fungus blastospores could be observed in the blood at 1000x magnification, there was some doubt that this was conclusive. The doubt was reported in the popular book "The Yeast Syndrome" by Trowbridge and Walker. However, over the year 1986, the evidence became much more conclusive, as the budding process was observed and the rhizoid tentacles seen invading cells. In June, 1987, the general consensus was that the dark-field screening process is accurate. The staining procedure shows beyond a doubt the candida/fungus in the blood according to the medical doctors who employ this technology.

This puts the visual detection of candidiasis into the communities where patients can see it for themselves and not have to rely on inaccurate lab tests, expensive antibody lab tests, and reporting delays.

Dark-field microscopy must be conducted by a trained, competent technician, as improper slide preparations create the appearance of conditions a person doesn't really have, such as platelet aggregation (a clumping together of the red blood cells). Properly prepared slides, however, are an excellent screening for a variety of nutritional conditions and serve to verify the effectiveness of the nutritional work at a later screening.

When a person can actually see the candida fungus in their blood it takes the guesswork out of the diagnosis. It also provides a strong visualization matrix for people interested in working mentally, as pioneered in cancer treatments, to remove the candida.

Electro-Acupuncture Evaluation

Electro-acupuncture is a health evaluation method that is becoming increasingly popular despite the reluctance of the "powers that be" to accept it. The work does not involve sticking needles into the body as some people think when they hear the word "acupuncture." It's simply a measurement of meridian energy pathways that leads to the ability to evaluate imbalances.

69

The first premise of electro-acupuncture is that everything is energy — rocks, plants, the human body, this book — are all composed of atoms or frequencies of energy.

In electro-acupuncture, diagnostic equipment very similar to an ohmmeter is used to measure the resistance in the body's acupuncture meridians. These meridians relate to the primary organs and tissues of the body.

For example, there is a liver meridian (as well as kidney, pancreas, circulatory, lymphatic, intestine, gall bladder, etc., meridians.) and any imbalance in the meridian measurement shows there is a problem, or a less than optimal state of health.

An examination with electro-acupuncture equipment means that the patient holds an electrode in one hand and the practitioner then presses various acupuncture points (usually on the hands and feet) with a probe. A meter registers the resistance on a dial or computer screen.

Since this is an energy-testing with electronic equipment, remedies or substances can be added to the circuit to see if their oscillations can correct an imbalance. With EAV equipment (Electro-Acupuncture-Voll — built and operated along the research lines of Dr. Reinhold Voll), the practitioner looks for an indicator drop on the meter. With EAP (Electro-Acupuncture) equipment, the practitioner looks for measurement values that fall outside the normal range. When an abnormal value is found, a remedy can be added to the circuit to see if it will restore the meter's indicator to the proper value. The oscillations of the remedy will show to correct the imbalance in the patient's meridian energy as viewed on the meter.

With electro-acupuncture equipment, the practitioner can determine which remedies (homeopathics, herbs, vitamins, minerals, glandular factors, extracts, foods, etc.) support the patient. A correctly chosen remedy contains the bio-magnetic field that helps the immune system correct the imbalance in the meridian energy. Since diseases first exist in the body's energy field before manifesting in the body, the energy field is an optimal area in which to work to restore health.

Here's an example: The practitioner tests the patient's intestinal meridian and finds an inflammatory reading. Then by adding substances to the circuit the search begins for the oscillations that will correct the problem. The first one chosen is an herb, golden seal, known for its anti-bacterial properties. The meter's indicator drops a few points, but does not enter the normal range. We now know that there is a little bacterial involvement, but that it is not the whole story. Next, a reversed-polarity pau d'arco extract known for its powerful antifungal properties is introduced. The meter's indicator locks into the normal range. Now we know that the problem in the intestine is fungal and we also know a good remedy.

To further check this, the practitioner puts a homeopathic nosode* of Candida albicans in the circuit. The response is good, but not quite where it should be. Next a homeopathic nosode* for Monilia albicans (a cousin of Candida) is put into the circuit and it once again locks into the normal range. Now we know the specific problem and two solutions. Putting both the pau d'arco extract and the nosode in the circuit shows that both work and both may be incorporated into the program. Now the patient has a custom-designed, energy-based program to restore a more optimal level of health.

Research by biochemist A.S. Wheelwright along these same lines has revealed some interesting concepts in energy-based nutrition. Wheelwright proposes that there are optimal levels at which every organ and tissue resonates. These patterns have several measurements that can be electronically determined. For instance, the kidney has a unique energy pattern based on its genetic blueprint. Since nutritional elements also have resonant patterns, he works to combine nutrients (herbs, vitamins, minerals, homeopathics, protomorphagens, cell salts, free-form amino acids, etc.) into energy patterns compatible with the designated organ or tissue's frequency and characteristics.

Many doctors and nutritionists working with Wheelwright's research believe that his work in energy-based nutrition is ushering in a new era in healing through nutrition.

Electro-acupuncture-type equipment is quite varied now that there are over 30 years of intensive research to build upon. Some of the various types are the Dermatron, Vega-test, MORA, Interro, and new state of the art Computron system, and there are many others.

71

Competence in electro-acupuncture comes with much study and practice. In competent hands, it is a powerful and excellent tool for the understanding of the factors that influence a person's health. As the primary tool of bio-energetic medicine, electro-acupuncture offers a safe and natural way to heal the body without the side effects caused by allopathic drugs.

Practiced openly by medical doctors in Europe, Canada, and many other parts of the world, this remarkable science has been withheld from the people of the United States by the combined interests of pharmaceutical manufacturers and their influence with the American Medical Association and the Food and Drug Administration. [Note: U.S. pharmaceutical companies are heavy investors in European homeopathic and biological medicines.] Safe and effective remedies are being withheld from the U.S. public along with their true healing powers, so the drug companies can make their profits. Someone needs to reaffirm that this is the land of the free. That responsibility rests with you and me.

ELECTRO-ACUPUNCTURE CHART

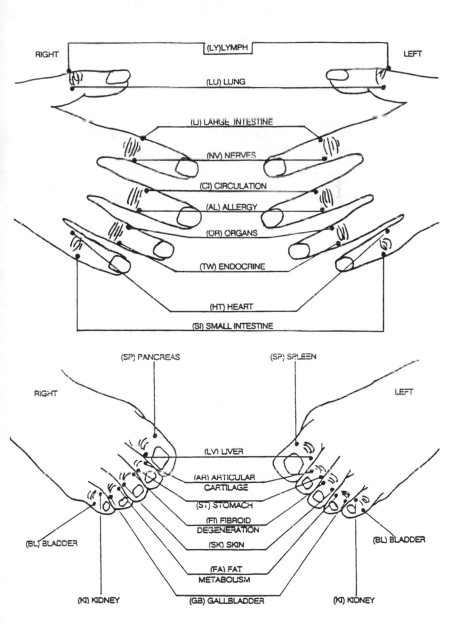

73

KINESIOLOGY/BIO-KINESIOLOGY

Since we've already explored electro-acupuncture, it's easy to say that kinesiology is very similiar in principle. Only the method is different. Instead of a meter, the muscle response is used as an indicator. This is why this science is called "muscle testing."

As with electro-acupuncture, weak meridians, organs, and tissues can be determined and appropriate remedies chosen. The circuit is made between the practitioner and the patient. A muscle, such as the deltoid, is tested for strength by pushing on the arm. A wide variety of muscles may be tested, as different muscles relate to different organ groups.

When a muscle responds to testing with normal strength, it indicates there is proper nerve supply. When a muscle responds with below normal strength, it indicates interference with normal nerve-system function. The validity of muscle testing has been well proven by EEG, EKG, and polygraph-type equipment.

Kinesiology, although a somewhat subjective science, is becoming more recognized and is sometimes taught in chiropractic colleges. Once again, in competent hands, kinesiology can help determine which area of the body needs support and what kind of support is required (structural, chemical, electromagnetic), what the dosage should be, and even the duration of treatment. It calls upon the body's innate wisdom and healing powers to determine the best course of action. The language of kinesiology can be interpreted by trained professionals who align themselves with an understanding of the body's connection with its life force and the natural laws that stem from that inherent wisdom.

DERMATOGLYPHICS

One of the most fascinating of the subjective evaluation methods involves the lines on the soles of the feet. A person has to know what to look for, but this unusual evaluation method developed by A. Stuart Wheelwright has proven itself again and again when blood tests are conducted after initially suspecting candida from the lines in the feet.

Wheelwright has discovered how to identify a dozen different kinds of candida/fungus by the fine lines and markings on the bottom of the feet. When more conclusive testing is done that shows the healing processes, he will allow this evaluation method to be printed. In the meantime it is taught to those attending seminars on Sclerology (interpreting the red lines in the white of the eyes) and dermatoglyphics (interpreting the lines on the soles of the feet). [For more information on classes and activities, contact the International Sclerology Foundation, 4201 Bee Caves Road, Suite C-212, Austin, Texas 78746.] Home study course available.

Many people have heard of a foot massage therapy called reflexology — a derivative of acupuncture, which presses and massages the sore nerve (meridian) endings on the bottom of the feet, thus freeing the energy-impeding crystals and fractured DNA molecules so the body can more readily heal itself. There are many books on reflexology available. If the candida-identifying lines appear over the pancreas or hip or colon zones as defined in reflexology, then candidiasis can be suspected to be disturbing that area.

On the next page is a standard map of the zones in the bottom of the feet.

REFLEX ZONE CHART

LEFT FOOT

Frontal Sinus
Temple

Right Eye
Right Ear
Levator Scapul Muscle
Shoulder
Heart
Adrenal Gland
Spleen
Colon Transversum
Colon Descendens
Left Knee
Rectum

Pituitary Body
Cerebrum
Nose
Medulla Oblongata, Cerebellum
Neck
Accessory Thyroid Gland
Thyroid Gland
Lung, Trachea
Solar Plexus
Stomach
Pancreas
Duodenum
Kidney
Ureter
Small Intestine
Bladder
Anus
Testis, Ovary

REFLEX ZONE CHART

RIGHT FOOT

Temple

Pituitary Body
Cerebrum
Nose
Medulla Oblongata, Cerebellum
Neck
Accessory Thyroid Gland
Thyroid Gland
Lung, Trachea
Solar Plexus
Stomach
Pancreas
Duodenum
Kidney
Ureter
Small Intestine
Bladder
Testis, Ovary

Frontal Sinus
Left Eye
Left Ear
Levator Scapulae Muscle
Right Shoulder
Liver
Gall Bladder
Adrenal Gland
Colon Transversum
Colon Ascendens
Ileum
Right Knee
Appendix

REFLEX ZONE CHART

76

Sclerology

The eye is a fabulous instrument! In addition to its remarkable ability to translate wavelengths of light into nerve impulses for vision, it registers the reflex nerve impulses from all over the body into a pattern that reveals specific stresses and conditions that are affecting a person's health.

The visible part of the eye has three sections — the pupil, the iris, and the SCLERA. A particularly revealing area to interpret is the sclera, or the white of the eye, as both the causative area and the affected area are revealed. The red lines on the white background of the sclera change as health conditions change, and appear in various shapes at different locations.

The science of the sclera — SCLEROLOGY — provides an understanding of the language of the eyes.

It is believed that these red lines provide information about abnormal stress conditions that exist at various locations in the body. These stresses can be anything from viral and bacterial infections, energy blockage, poor metabolism, nervous difficulties, poor circulation, congestions, degenerations, pH imbalances, parasitic involvement, to extreme abnormal conditions.

A unique feature of the sclera is that its line patterns may register an abnormal stress development long before any serious effects are experienced. This information may then be compared with other health-science evaluations, such as applied or bio-kinesiology, dermatoglyphics (reflex lines in the feet), and iridology, etc., to confirm this situation.

As the evaluations and interpretations are made, and the stress conditions understood, proper corrective measures can be applied. The body can then more easily adjust and alleviate the abnormal stresses, resulting in a greater degree of health.

To help you understand sclerology, the following premises are provided:

1. The eyes are indeed "the mirror of soul." They reveal changes, stresses, congestions, and abnormal conditions within the body.

2. The condition of every organ and part of the body is reflected in a specific area of the eye. The nerve filaments, muscle

fibers, and minute blood vessels in different areas of the eye portray the changing conditions in the corresponding parts and organs of the body.

3. The veins in the sclera reveal the disease process by their configurations, color, and placement. Proper evaluation reveals the cause of the distress.

4. The eye reveals, from the beginning, subtle changes in vital parts and organs, thus enabling a person to avert any threatening disease by correcting the causative factors nutritionally and other natural ways. The eye also shows the cleansing and healing processes, as the body adjusts to a more optimum state of health.

5. The eye contains an immense number of nerve filaments, which are connected to and receive reflective impressions from all areas of the body through the optic nerve, sympathetic nervous system, optic thalmi, and the spinal cord.

6. Sclerology enables the evaluator to ascertain from the appearance of the eye the person's predispostion to health and disease, the general constitution, the status of each individual organ, as well as each organ's and gland's influence on the other body systems.

Sclerology, combined with sound nutritional knowledge and application, can provide people the ability to consciously support their health and longevity, overcome and alleviate stresses, and live a more healthful life.

Although the lines in the feet are an initial indicator of the possibility of fungal involvement, some other clues may be found in the red lines of the whites of the eyes. The International Sclerology Foundation has compiled this information based on over 600 case histories. Although not conclusive as of July, 1988, the indicators given here could lead one to suspect candidiasis and thus seek verification by using other methods.

Below is the chart compiled by the International Sclerology Foundation based on the work of A. S. Wheelwright.

SCLEROLOGY

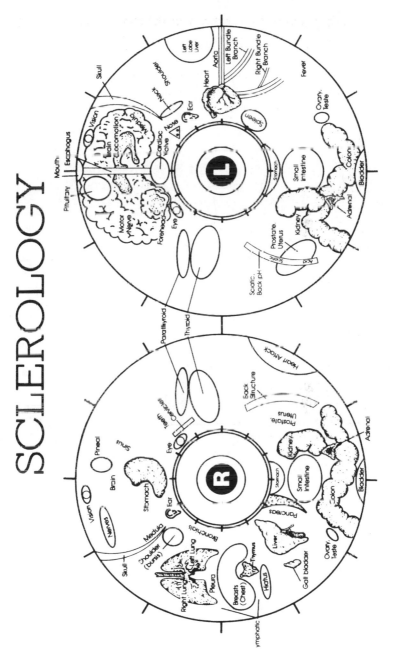

Copies of this chart (9 x 12") are available from the International Sclerology Foundation.

79

Sclerology clues to suspecting candidiasis.

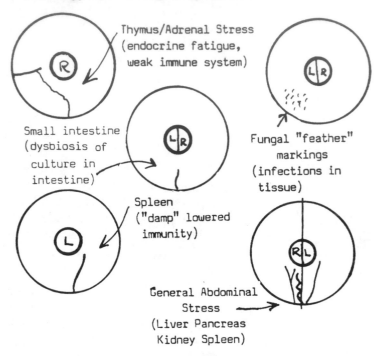

Dietary Diagnosis

Another method of suspecting candidiasis is by voluntarily putting yourself on a candida diet for a week to ten days followed by a period of including all the things you abstained from. Just see how you feel for a clue. This isn't very conclusive, yet many people are interested in experimenting with diet.

For instance, stop your intake of the major offenders, such as beer, wine, apple cider vinegar, fruit, bread, alfalfa sprouts (unless you first soak them in 1% hydrogen peroxide to kill off the molds), cheese, and all sugars for a week. This means that your diet will be basically vegetables and protein (fresh ocean fish, organic chicken, seeds, eggs, and so forth) with a minimum amount of complex carbohydrate (potatoes, rice, millet, yams, etc.). This isn't such a bad idea anyway, as it is a vast improvement over what is considered the Standard American Diet promoted by the food lobbies and supported by the A.M.A. and dieticians.

For example, for breakfast have 75% vegetables (mostly raw, some lightly cooked) with a small yard egg omlet, and soaked seeds (sesame, sunflower, pumpkin). For lunch have a large salad, steamed vegetables and a piece of fish. For supper, have soup and a salad. This would be the time for a little complex carbohydrate such as some rice or a couple of new potatoes. This is basically what all the books say to eat as the standard candida diet.

Some words of caution: If this method of eating is a radical departure from your current diet — one heavy on the fast foods, candies, red meats, and desserts — the dietary change alone can cause a cleansing reaction that can cause many toxins to dump out of the tissues into the bloodstream to be removed from the body. (Freed from dietary stress, the body has the energy to cleanse itself.) If this were to occur, you would feel worse than ever, but it is the natural pathway to health. The best recommendation as you begin such a program is that you obtain the help of a professional nutritionist.

Eat this way for a week or ten days. Then revert back to your old diet, which includes the offenders. Have a beer, eat sugar and desserts, enjoy bread. How do you feel? If your energy drops, allergies flare up, and other symptoms of candidiasis show up, then you have a pretty good idea that candida is a problem. And you have a pretty good idea how to control it through diet.

Questionnaires

There are a couple of questionnaires designed to measure the possibility of candida involvement.

The first one, "The Candida Score Sheet," has been floating around for quite a while. I think it was developed by Dr. Crook and then circulated by hundreds of different companies. It is made available here as it is the most widely used questionnaire.

The second one, the "Candidiasis Potential Appraisal," is called "the short form". We developed it in 1985 to provide initial screening and save time, as patients are traditionally bombarded with questionnaires when they seek professional nutritional advice.

Candida Questionnaire
And Score Sheet

This questionnaire is designed for adults and the scoring system isn't appropriate for children. It lists factors in your medical history which promote the growth of candida albicans (Section A), and symptoms commonly found in individuals with yeast-connected illness (Sections B and C).

For each "Yes" answer in Section A, circle the point score in that section. Record your total score in the box at the end of the section. Then move on to Sections B and C and score as directed.

Filling out and scoring this questionnaire should help you and your doctor evaluate the possible role of candida in contributing to your health problems. Yet it will not provide an automatic "Yes" or "No" answer.

Section A: History

Point Score

1. Have you taken tetracyclines (Symycin®, Panmycin®, Vibramycin®, Minocin®, etc.) or other antibiotics for acne for one month or longer? 25

2. Have you, at any time in your life, taken other "broad spectrum" antibiotics* for respiratory, urinary or other infections for 2 months or longer or in shorter courses 4 or more times in a 1-year period? 20

3. Have you taken a broad spectrum antibiotic* — even in a single course? 6

4. Have you, at any time in your life, been bothered by persistent prostatitis, vaginitis or other problems affecting your reproductive organs? 25

5. Have you been pregnant...
   2 or more times? 5
   1 time? 3

*Including Keflex®, ampicillin, amoxicillin, Ceclor®, Bactrim®, and Septra®. Such antibiotics kill off "good germs" while they are killing off those which cause infection.

6. Have you taken birth control pills...
   For more than 2 years? 15
   For 6 months to 2 years? 8
7. Have you taken prednisone, Decadron
   or other cortisone-type drugs...
   For more than 2 weeks? 15
   For 2 weeks or less? 6
8. Does exposure to perfumes, insecti-
   cides, fabric shop odors and other
   chemicals provoke...
   Moderate to severe symptoms? 20
   Mild Symptoms? 5
9. Are your symptoms worse on damp,
   muggy days or in moldy places? 20
10. Have you had athlete's foot, ring
    worm, jock itch or other chronic fun-
    gus infections of the skin or nails?
    Have such infections been...
    Severe or persistent? 20
    Mild to to moderate? 10
11. Do you crave sugar? 10
12. Do you crave breads? 10
13. Do you crave alcoholic beverages? 10
14. Does tobacco smoke really bother you? . 10

Total Score, Section A   _____

Section B: Major Symptoms
For each of your symptoms, enter the appropriate figure in the point score column:

Occasional or mild . . . . 3 points

Frequent and/or moderately severe 6 points

Severe and/or disabling . . . . 9 points

Add total score and record it in the box at the
end of this section: Point Score

1. Fatigue or lethargy   _____
2. Feeling of being "drained"   _____
3. Poor memory   _____
4. Feeling "spacey" or "unreal"   _____
5. Depression   _____
6. Numbness, burning or tingling   _____
7. Muscle Aches   _____
8. Muscle weakness or paralysis   _____
9. Pain and/or swelling in joints   _____

83

10. Abdominal pain _____

11. Constipation _____

12. Diarrhea _____

13. Bloating _____

14. Troublesome vaginal discharge _____

15. Persistent vaginal burning or itching _____

16. Prostatitis _____

17. Impotence _____

18. Loss of sexual desire _____

19. Endometriosis _____

20. Cramps and/or other menstrual irregularities _____

21. Premenstrual tension _____

22. Spots in front of the eyes _____

23. Erratic vision _____

Total Score, Section B _____

Section C: Other Symptoms

For each of your symptoms, enter the appropriate figure in the point score column:

Occasional or mild . . . . 1 point
Frequent and/or moderately severe 2 points
Severe and/or disabling . . . . 3 points

Add total score and record it in the box at the end of this section.

Point Score

1. Drowsiness _____

2. Irritability or jitteriness _____

3. Incoordination _____

4. Inability to concentrate _____

5. Frequent mood swings _____

6. Headache _____

7. Dizziness/loss of balance _____

8. Pressure above ears, feeling of head swelling and tingling _____

9. Itching _____

10. Other rashes _____

11. Heartburn _____

12. Indigestion _____

13. Belching and intestinal gas _____

14. Mucus in stools _____

15. Hemorrhoids _____

84

16. Dry mouth	_____
17. Rash or blisters in mouth	_____
18. Bad breath	_____
19. Joint swelling or arthritis	_____
20. Nasal congestion or discharge	_____
21. Postnasal drip	_____
22. Nasal itching	_____
23. Sore or dry throat	_____
24. Cough	_____
25. Pain or tightness in chest	_____
26. Wheezing or shortness of breath	_____
27. Urinary urgency or frequency	_____
28. Burning on urination	_____
29. Failing vision	_____
30. Burning or tearing of eyes	_____
31. Recurrent infections or fluid in ears	_____
32. Ear pain or deafness	_____
Total Score, Section C	_____
Total Score, Section A	_____
Total Score, Section B	_____
GRAND TOTAL SCORE	_____

The Grand Total Score will help you and your doctor decide if your health problems are yeast-connected. Scores in women will run higher as 7 items in the questionnaire apply exclusively to women, while only 2 apply exclusively to men.

If your score is:	Symptoms are:
180 (women) 140 (men)	Almost Certainly Yeast Connected
120 (women) 90 (men)	Probably Yeast Connected
60 (women) 40 (men)	Possibly Yeast Connected
Less Than 60 (women) 40 (men)	Probably Not Yeast Connected

CANDIDIASIS POTENTIAL APPRAISAL

Questionnaires such as this can provide insights into the possibility that candidiasis may be a factor in your health. It cannot provide conclusive evidence, but high-scorers are encouraged to get more information.

HISTORY (Circle the points if the question applies.)
POINTS

1. Were you breast-fed as an infant? If not, ... 9

2. Have you ever had a broad-spectrum antibiotic?

    A single course, or 4

    A month or longer 9

3. Antibiotics more than 3 times in one year? 9

4. Have you taken cortisone drugs (Prednisone)? 5

5. Do you have fungal infections (athlete's foot, fungus under toenails, jock itch)? 7

6. Are symptoms worse on rainy, muggy days, or if in moldy areas (cellars, leaf piles)? 7

7. Do you crave:

    sugar, sweets 5

    alcohol (beer, wine, distilled spirits) 4

    carbohydrates (breads)? 5

8. Are you sensitive to:

    tobacco smoke 3

    perfumes 3

    insecticides, chemical odors? 3

9. Women only:

    A. Persistent or recurring vaginitis? 9

    B. Any pregnancies? 3

    C. Take birth control pills? 9

SYMPTOMS
(rate: mild — 1 pt., moderate — 2 pts., severe — 3 pts.)

10. Constipation/diarrhea .... ____

11. Bloating, gas .... ____

12. Tired, lethargic, drained .... ____

13. Poor memory, spacey, unable to concentrate .... ____

14. Depression, mood swings .... ____

15. Burning, tingling, numbness .... ____

16 Muscle aches, weakness, pain in joints .... ____

17. Women: troublesome vaginal discharge, burning .... ____
    Men: prostatitis, impotence, urinary burning .... ____

18. Abdominal pain .... ____

19. Spots in front of eyes, vision fading .... ____

20. Women: premenstrual syndrome, severe cramps .... ____
    Men: frequent rashes in groin area .... ____

21. Cold hands and feet .... ____

                                          TOTAL _____

Scoring:

   Scores over 32 for women, and over 28 for men indicate that
Candidiasis could play a major part in your symptoms.

TREATMENTS OF CANDIDIASIS

To truly conquer candida, a carefully thought-out strategy must be employed. We'll discuss this in the section called "A Plan To Conquer Candida," but to understand the strategy, let's first take a look at what's being done so far. Now that candidiasis has been pandemic for several years, many things have been tried, and we now have the perspective of hindsight, as well as knowing what's currently helping.

To date, treatment of candidiasis has focused on killing yeast and fungus, with only occasional focus on preventing its recurrence and virtually nothing being done to restore the immune system. The closest thing to a complete strategy has come through the alternative medicine and nutrition field. Orthodox medicine has been limited in creating a comprehensive plan primarily because such a plan would have to include nutrition. Let's take a look at current treatments — their scope, effectiveness, and failures, as verified by clinical experience with over 600 people during a 3 1/2-year period.

The Drug Nystatin

The medical approach to candidiasis is to kill yeast and fungus with the antibiotic-type drug nystatin and to keep giving it until somehow the patient gets better. This therapy works fairly well, and in cases of severe dysbiosis*, it is critically important to kill the candida before it eats a person alive. If necessary, nystatin can be used in extreme cases, and then more nutritionally-oriented steps can be taken in hopes of a complete turn around.

Nystatin works by attaching itself to the cell wall of yeasts, which increases the permeability of the membrane and thus allows the cellular material to spill out, resulting in death of the cell. By reducing the constant presence of yeasts and thus unlocking the immunologic tolerance, it is hoped the body can once again fight yeast on its own and restore its own health.

It's important to realize that drugs do not cure. And nystatin does not cure. It only kills candida in the G.I. tract and vaginal area if used topically, in hopes the immune system can make a comeback and a person can regain health. This is typical of all antibiotic therapy. If nystatin can kill the candida and the immune system can recover, then the therapy is considered successful.

There's something very odd about using an antibiotic to help a person recover from the devastating effects of past antibiotic use. Nonetheless, this is the best medical science has to offer at this time. For those who cannot tolerate nystatin, the drug ketoconazole (Nizoral) is often used as an antifungal agent, although it is not as specific as nystatin. Also, ketoconazole can cause serious liver damage. Close supervision by a doctor is required. Ketoconazole cannot work for patients with immune suppressive disorders as it requires active white blood cells for success.

Nystatin is not effective for all types of fungus. It is very specific, and many types of cell-invasive fungus are resistant to it. Another limitation is that, like penicillin, nystatin is a mold (fungus/bacteria) by-product — a derivative of Streptomyces noursei. People who are sensitive to molds and have reactions to them may be reactive to nystatin.

One other concern — a major one — is that microorganisms are very adaptable, and nystatin may well be creating nystatin-resistant strains. This has happened with other antibiotics, so it's the same old story. Nature shows us again and again that most drugs are not in accord with natural law. Yet there are antibiotic-type herbs that help eliminate the organisms, but do not allow them to build up a tolerance, because their action is to support the immune response rather than just kill bacteria.

Sometimes when an antibiotic such as tetracycline is required, a doctor may also prescribe the antifungal drug Amphotericin-B to offset the candida caused by the antibiotic. Amphotericin-B's side effects include liver damage and nervous disorders. It is a very toxic substance.

Nystatin Overview
• Specific antibiotic for candida
• Allows other fungi to proliferate (trichophyton)
• Does not control candida in the blood or tissue
• May be encouraging new, more resistant strains
• Must be repeated often and used for lengthy duration (years).

Nystatin has helped many a person regain their health and has actually saved lives, but the results are often only temporary, and the treatment must be repeated. It is not uncommon for people to take nystatin for six months and then have to begin again because they have a flare up as soon as the drug is discontinued. As I said, nystatin does not cure. Only the body can cure itself, and only when the cause is corrected. We know the cause is dysbiosis in the G.I. tract combined with a weakened immune system.

On the natural side, several herbs, vitamins, and treatments have emerged to be effective often in controlling candida.

Antigen Stimulation (Vaccine Therapy)

Some doctors treat candidiasis as they would allergies — with injections of the diluted offender. Just as dilutions of ragweed are given as "allergy shots" to people with sensitivities to ragweed, shots of diluted Candida albicans are given to people with suspected candidiasis.

This treatment is based upon the fact that people suffering from candidiasis have immune systems that are unresponsive to the candida antigens. Their body's begin to accept candida as "self" and no longer fight it. This is based on the presence of thymus-derived T-suppressor cells, which specifically inhibit the immune system's response to candida due to chronic exposure. The purpose of the shots is to restore the immune system's response to candida antigens.

Antigenic stimulation therapy is somewhat experimental, as different types of candida extracts are needed. Testing is done by the skin "scratch test" method where an injection of extract is observed for immediate or delayed reaction (wheal).

Results with candida injections have been similar to allergy shot treatments — some successes, some failures. The injections of candida extracts attempt to strengthen the immune response, but there is quite a bit of inconsistency in results. It has not been possible to standardize the program, due to the wide variety of types of candida and the many varied reactions of people affected by it. The strength of the extract, the time factor between treatments, the individual nature of the patient's immune response, the type of extract, and the extent of the patient's immune system deficiency all have a bearing on the results.

Results with this type of experimental therapy have been hard-won. Each patient's program is arbitrary, and adjustments must be made based on the patient's response. There is a lot of guesswork and much room for error. Such therapy does not, of itself, treat the cause.

Candidiasis is complex because it is both an infection and an allergic response to the byproducts of yeast/fungus metabolism.

Pau d'Arco

Pau d'arco (also called taheebo, ipe roxo, and la pacho) is a South American herb with proven antifungal properties. In Brazil it is used as a treatment for cancer, diabetes, and a host of other diseases, although results in North America have not shown it to be effective for such serious diseases.

In the Amazon basin there is fungus on practically every plant — except a tree whose bark stays clean and shiny. This tree is called "la pacho" (pau d'arco). Its inner bark has powerful antifungal properties.

In the early 1980s this herb became popular in the United States as a panacea — a cure-all for everything. As the demand for pau d'arco increased, the quality decreased. It became a big business with the usual dealings of middle men, the dilution of the product, and so forth. Instead of importing the potent inner bark, companies began importing the shredded up outer bark mixed with the inner bark. This gave more bulk, a lower cost, and higher profits. It did not give good results. Also as the demand increased, rumors of Brazilian use of Agent Orange (2-4-5-T) to defoliate the jungle became a concern to many health-minded people.

Other sources of pau d'arco (ipe roxo variety) were located in Peru so some of the smaller companies and research labs still use a good quality herb in their products.

By the mid 1980s people were drinking pau d'arco tea out the ears, but not getting the incredible, medically-documented results that were obtained in Brazil. This puzzled Stuart Wheelwright. In his studies with herbs he learned that herbs grown south of the equator worked differently when used north of the equator. He attributed this to the difference in molecular rotation (magnetic field) between the northern and southern hemispheres.

91

He observed that water going down a drain in South America turns counterclockwise, whereas in North America it turns clockwise. This natural rotation of the magnetic field of the Earth affects the plants grown there. Wheelwright wondered if this rotation could be the reason for pau d'arco's inability to work as well as it should when used by northern hemisphere inhabitants, whose body systems, he felt, were more accustomed to elements derrived in a clockwise magnetic field.

Using equipment called a microcycletron (the same kind of equipment Eastman Kodak uses to turn synthetic vitamin E into "natural" vitamin E by reversing the synthetic's molecular rotation), he reversed the molecular rotation of pau d'arco and found it then to be quite incredible from an energy perspective. He later began to manufacture small batches of reversed-polarity extract of pau d'arco (combined with the herbs cynita and ceriece) for an even greater synergistic effect. He called it "Tai Ra Chi."

This extract brings the full power of pau d'arco's antifungal properties to bear in the northern hemisphere. The research book Candida, Silver (Mercury) Fillings, and the Immune System by Betsy Russell-Manning was the first publication to present this extract as the true essence of what pau d'arco was supposed to do — strengthen the immune system, kill fungus and inhibit its growth.

In any case, pau d'arco as a tea is not very effective unless a lot (three quarts) were to be used each day. It's just not strong enough to tackle a full-blown case of candidiasis. And since pau d'arco is a diuretic (promotes the removal of water by urination), excessive use in tea form can deplete vital minerals such as sodium, potassium, calcium, magnesium, and trace minerals. So additional supplementation is required for therapeutic tea use. Pau d'arco extracts work much better, because they are more concentrated and do not upset the mineral balance.

Three drops of the reversal polarity extract accomplish what the three quarts of pau d'arco tea can, as verified by measuring fungus residues in the bloodstream using dark-field microscopy.

Note: As with nystatin, any natural antifungal can cause a die-off reaction as it kills the toxic fungus. Even the natural antifungals should be used sparingly at first, to see if a die-off reaction occurs, and gradually built up as the overall toxic level is decreased.

If a die-off reaction occurs, a person should use a hydrogogue laxative to encourage an enthusiastic bowel elimination. This is one that promotes the movement of water into the bowel rather than just irritating the bowel to empty. The movement of water into the bowel carries the toxins with it for more rapid recovery. Kidney support is also required, as is additional water intake, to flush out the toxins should a "die off" reaction occur.

Pau d'arco does not reach the deep tissue in most cases. It is not a cure, but it plays an important role in conquering candidiasis by helping the body get rid of candida without suppressing the immune system. Its particular forte seems to be eliminating fungus from the bloodstream. It is typical to find the blood completely clean of fungus after two to four weeks use of the reversed polarity pau d'arco extract mentioned above.

Garlic

You may have noticed that there's quite a bit being said about garlic lately. It has proven itself over the years to be an effective antibiotic, and its active ingredient, allicin, is fairly successful in killing candida. Most of the "deodorized" garlic has the allicin removed so it is NOT able to function as an antibiotic/antifungal. A few manufacturers of garlic supplements have learned how to deodorize it and retain the antifungal properties. This allows people to use large quantities and maintain a social life. If you choose to supplement with garlic, be sure it contains its active ingredient, allicin.

Garlic may be used fresh or odorless as found in supplemental capsules. One concern nutritionists are having regarding garlic is that some of it is being irradiated as a preservative method. Garlic is not an all-purpose antifungal as it can get moldy itself. Food irradiation is a controversial topic in that nuclear wastes are used to gamma-radiate foods to rid them of parasites, preserve them, and lengthen their shelf life.

Unfortunately, unknown particles are created by this process, and no one knows the impact they will have. Although there's no detectable radiation left on the food, the life force is destroyed. The food cannot sprout. Its enzymes are killed and enzymes are by far the most important nutrient in food. It also resists molding and spoiling. Irradiated garlic no longer contains its power to kill fungus. At a time when people need all the life-force they can get from their food, using dead food that's been irradiated only contributes to the disease processes.

So if the garlic you use has been irradiated (and due to bureaucratic red tape it probably will not be labeled as such), it will not help you much with fighting candida. It's best to grow your own or seek out garlic that is still alive — the kind that will sprout. As far as I know, the reputable companies that put out a garlic supplement use only fresh, living garlic.

Garlic does not cure candidiasis. Advertising in the health field often tries to push the limits of what legally can be said (that is the way of advertising). This is important to understand. A new push to market garlic as a cure-all is underway. Garlic can help with many health conditions, including cardiovascular problems and infections. A number of in vitro* and in vivo* studies of allicin's antifungal properties are being documented, so it's a viable adjunct to a candidiasis program.

In the same antibacterial category with garlic are other herbs — onion, aloe, horseradish, and clove (eugenol). Garlic can help, but it is not the answer as some of the advertising suggests.

Garlic is a wonderful, nutritious herb that may contain the mineral germanium whch we'll discuss later. Including it in your diet is a practical and beneficial idea provided you are not allergic to it.

Chlorolphyll

Chlorophyll is the green, photosynthesis-activated part of plants, known for years as a wonder food — one that cleanses, nourishes, and heals the body. Its chemical components are almost identical to that of human red blood. In concentrated amounts, it is known to inhibit bacteria and relieve many of the discomforts of candidiasis — itching, burning, gas, bloating.

Chlorophyll can break the carbon dioxide molecule (CO_2) and release the oxygen (O_2), thus providing an environment that inhibits the proliferation of detrimental anaerobic bacteria.

It is not a cure for candida, but it is a valuable step in the direction of the good nutrition people are lacking. It is also an intestional cleanser that helps restore normal bacteria culture.

Many people use wheatgrass juice as a source of concentrated chlorophyll. This is valuable but it contains a lot of sugar, which may aggravate the condition of people with candidiasis. Rye grass and barley grass test to be better sources — they are lower in sugar and have been less tampered with by humans. The inbred smut-resistant factor in wheat has genetically altered the plant, making it far more allergenic than it was prior to 1926.

From a nutritional standpoint, additional chlorophyll in the diet is a tremendous step toward health. Include more green vegetables and/or use supplements such as Green Magma , Barley Green , Greenlife , chlorella, alfalfa, etc., to increase your supply of this valuable nutritional booster.

Biotin

The B vitamin, biotin, plays a role in fighting candida in that the conversion of the yeast to its fungal form occurs best in a biotin deficient environment. Supplementing with biotin can prevent the conversion of yeast to the cell-invasive fungus.

Should you want to supplement your diet with biotin, find a natural, yeast-free, 300-microgram source and use it throughout the day, with and away from food. That's approximately 7 to 10 doses.

Keep in mind that B vitamins work as a team with other members of the B-complex family, as well as other nutrients. Imbalances can occur when one B vitamin is taken alone.

We learn from Nature that no vitamins exist independently. They all are present with other synergists. If you supplement with biotin, be sure to include a complete, yeast-free, B-complex supplement to provide other B-vitamin factors. Too much of any vitamin is unnecessarily stimulating and stressful to the body.

Biotin also works to build certain antibodies. You might want to consider foods that are rich in biotin as well. This way your intake includes natural biotin as it occurs in foods. Supplemental biotin is usually synthetic. Rich sources of biotin include: egg yolk (cook at low temperature — 180-200 degrees F), organic calve's liver, whole grains, cauliflower, and legumes.

Biotin is produced by the beneficial intestinal bacteria — the ones missing when antibiotics kill off the flora. It also works with zinc and may have a relationship with the mineral germanium — both of which support the immune system. So you can see how one thing leads to another. Damage the beneficial bacteria and the immune system is damaged. Candida further stresses the immune system, and around it goes, all the way into chronic degenerative diseases.

Arginine (Free-Form Amino Acid)

Some nutritionists recommend free-form arginine to stimulate the thymus and its production of T-cells. Although arginine does activate the thymus, there are a number of contraindications that make taking it a foolhardy experiment.

Use of single free-form amino acids can be dangerous and should be considered as risky as drug therapy. Single amino acids do not occur in nature. Like vitamins and minerals, they occur along with factors — synergists — that enhance or buffer whatever the individual action may be. The general rule of safety regarding nutritional use of amino acids is that they should always be used in combinations of three or more — and preferably all. Unless an amino acid profile lab test is conducted to determine deficiencies and excesses, taking a single amino acid is risky. Use of a single amino acid can cause imbalances in the other amino acids, as they attempt to adjust to body-defined metabolism.

In free form, arginine enhances herpes simplex and herpes progenitalis infection causing outbreaks of lesions. It can also cause rough, coarse skin on knees, tops of toes, and elbows.

Homeopathy and Homeopathic Specifics

For an introduction to homeopathy and how it works we'll use excerpts from Cecil Craig's article, "Homeopathy, what it is, how it works."

"Homeopathy is a therapeutic system of medicine developed by Dr. Samuel Hahnemann over 170 years ago in Germany. Since that time it has spread to every country of the world. It is based upon the law of similars — 'like cures like symptoms.' This means that a substance given in large crude dosages will produce specific symptoms, but when this same material has been reduced in size and administered in minute doses, it will stimulate the body's reactive processes to remove these same symptoms. An example is Ipecacuanha (Ipecac). If taken in large quantities it produces vomiting, but taken in minute doses it cures vomiting. It will even stop the gagging which frequently follows a coughing spell when administered in minute Homeopathic amounts."

"There are over 2000 Homeopathic remedies. Furthermore, new substances are being added in Europe and Asia every day to cope with the new problems which arise in modern civilization. In normal practice probably less than half of the total list are ever indicated, and most practitioners utilize only 200 or 300 remedies on a regular basis. However, since most common remedies treat many conditions, an enormous amount of knowledge and professional training are required in the practice of Homeopathy."

"The Homeopathic practitioner studies his patients in great detail. His aim is to know and treat the whole person not just a single organ, and his "patient history" is of necessity far more detailed than most. After a careful consideration of the background and current symptoms, he is usually able to select the exact remedy for the individual. Where no such doctor is available, however, the layman can utilize a combination of three or four remedies which have been proven individually to apply to the symptoms he feels and this gives a better chance of getting the right remedy quickly. It should be remembered, though, that when the illness has persisted for years and become chronic, it may take more time to achieve results."

"Any substance might be used Homeopathically but most of these remedies are natural substances made from vegetable, animal, and mineral sources which are broken down into minute quantities to stimulate the natural defenses of the body. They do not cover up or stifle a symptom, and it may take time before the patient begins to feel better. But the patient's own defenses, properly stimulated, are usually sufficient to return him to health. In a combination any single remedy which does not cause such a reactive process will be passed off as a minute amount of natural substance. For this reason Homeopathic remedies are perfectly safe to take.

"Many Allopathic medicines are administered with the intent of destroying a specific disease organism. At the same time these drugs may be destroying beneficial bacteria often creating side effects which cause as much harm as the original problem. Other drugs palliate or cover up the symptoms and with sensitive individuals can actually poison the entire system. Drug induced reactions are becoming so prevalent that the government agencies require that all such drugs carry an insert telling about their possible harmful reactions. Homeopathic remedies neither cover up nor destroy disease by themselves. They stimulate the body's reaction to throw off the offender. Hence they do not create the side effects of many regular drugs, and no warnings or cautions are required on Homeopathic remedies beyond the standard 'if symptoms persist or increase in severity, consult a physician.'"

"Homeopathy, with its single purpose of attention to the whole human being and the prescribing of the simple remedy to trigger the VITAL FORCE within the human constitution to begin its own curative process, is a medical philosophy which is being recognized and extensively used by physicians throughout the world."

From the standpoint of classical homeopathy, the right fundamental remedy would boost a person's constitution to a level where it is able to overcome the ailments and symptoms that are exhibited. A fundamental remedy does not treat candida, it treats the individual's constitution. Once stimulated, the vital force of the individual is called upon to adjust the candidiasis imbalance as best it can. Such a remedy cannot replace lost culture in the G.I. tract, but it can promote, for a period of time, an immunological response to help a person overcome candidiasis.

From the standpoint of specific homeopathic remedies for candidiasis, there are several to consider. Borax is the standard remedy for thrush (aphthae), followed by Natrum Mur. Also, potentizations of candida itself are used. This is called "nosode" therapy, which involves the expectation that a diluted/potentized candida or monilia will trigger an immune response and help a person overcome the candida involvement.

The nosode posts "wanted posters" for the immune system, so the body knows exactly what to do. The immune system's confusion is temporarily clarified and an appropriate response solicited.

The usual procedure with nosodes is to start with a low potency, such as 5x or 6x, and gradually increase to high potencies, such as 200x or 1000x.

This treatment has proven itself clinically to be around 38% effective, making it a valuable tool. Its effectiveness is greatly enhanced by the addition of reversed-polarity pau d'arco and other nutritional supports.

A word of caution is needed regarding nosode therapy for candidiasis. In some cases it has been found to drive the candida in deeper, rather than drive it completely out of the body. The nosodes definitely harness an immunological response, but perhaps candida has a mind of its own and flees into deep tissue as well as out of the body. For this reason, the nosode program is greatly enhanced by simultaneous application of anti-candida nutritional therapies, particularly as outlined in the Wheelwright research known as "#4 (Corrector) [See your health professional] which serves as a drainage remedy to ensure the candida moves from the cells to the toilet bowl, rather than escaping to reappear when the therapy is discontinued.

Nosode therapy is best handled by professional nutritionists and doctors with a thorough background in homeopathy who have the ability to tell when a person should change potencies and who know how to accommodate the drainage of the candida from the body via a "drainage" remedy.

The German research on nosodes teaches that they should always be administered with an accompanying "drainage" remedy. An example is Berberis if drainage is conducted through the kidneys. Other drainage remedies are chosen if the liver, bowel, sinus, or skin is involved. The Hobon "Detoxosode" remedy is a broad-application drainage remedy.

The main difficulties in nosode treatments in the U.S. come from the product marketing companies, which give doctors questionnaires and protocols to follow that help them sell their nosode products. Doctors, chiropractors, and osteopaths not well-versed in homeopathy (it was not taught in school) proceed to treat their patients with nosodes as the "cure all" based on what the sales literature says, rather than on sound homeopathic principles. The determining factor seems to be: did the doctor learn nosode therapy by studying homeopathy, or did the doctor learn it from a company's sales rep? Fortunately, most biological medicines "do no harm," so risk to the patient is minimized if a remedy is not appropriate.

Nosode therapy has helped many people and continues to be a valuable natural therapy in helping people recover from candidiasis - a valuable part of a comprehensive program.

Aloe Vera

Just when it seemed that the juice from this healing, desert plant had been over-touted and multi-level marketed to death, some genuine benefits for candida patients began to emerge — particularly for those whose stomachs are so sensitive they can hardly eat or take nutritional supplements. Aloe vera does indeed have mild anti-candida properties. It can help reduce yeasts in the G.I. tract and promote beneficial bacteria.

This anti-candida action does not seem to carry over into the blood or tissue, so it is in no way a cure for candidiasis. It may help some — particularly when the stomach is oversensitive.

Note: You must use a high-quality aloe vera juice or use the gel from your own plants — not the green, outer leaf.

The thick skin (outer leaf) tests to be toxic. Many aloe vera companies simply juice the whole leaf, including the toxic outer skin. This results in a bitter liquid which is then "stabilized". The outer leaf does contain more beneficial mucopolysaccharides, but they are accompanied with undesirable elements.

Juice from the inner pulp is not bitter. It is often sold without other flavoring or treatments.

Based on the research of Dr. Clyde Johnson (one of the world's foremost skin chemistry experts), aloe vera does not seem to be the cure-all some companies claim. The oil does not break down to the cellular level. For this reason, it is excellent for burns as it coats the skin, but it is not really "food" for the skin cells since it is molecularly too large. So for burns and ulcers where a coating action is beneficial, aloe vera excels. For cosmetics and shampoo, it doesn't promote genuine health because of the same clogging or coating action. For Candidiasis patients with hypersensitive stomachs, it can be the first step to tolerating nutritional therapies.

If you are considering buying an aloe vera product, look for high quality, pure inner gel.

Minerals: Zinc, Germanium, Selenium

Some minerals play a role in combating candida, but once again, exercise caution in taking a lot of any single mineral. Like vitamins, minerals work in relationship with other minerals. To increase one often decreases another and drives yet a third one higher. If you supplement individual minerals, always include a multiple mineral based on a balanced natural source such as sea water, inland sea beds, or sea vegetation such as Irish moss, dulse, kelp, bladderwrack, etc. This will provide a broad mineral base to support the ones on which you are capitalizing.

The primary function of the anti-candida minerals is to support the immune system (e.g., the antioxidant action of zinc protects the body from free radicals).

Recent studies by Boyne and Arthur show selenium deficiencies to be involved with lowered resistance to candida.

Germanium, a trace mineral also known as vitamin O, has interesting potential as support for the immune system. A relatively new discovery, this age-old nutrient is found in many of the wonder foods and may, in fact, contribute greatly to the healing qualities of such wonder foods as ginseng (particularly Siberian and Red American), garlic, kelp, dulse, Irish moss, aloe vera, chlorella, watercress, and comfrey. (Avoid using comfrey if cancerous activity is occuring, as it is a cell-proliferent.)

Be wary of germanium capsule peddlers' claims that there's no toxic level and people can take all they want. This is contrary to the law of balance, and whether or not a lot of germanium makes people sick, too much of any good thing is always detrimental. (Even pure water can be drunk to excess and cause hallucinations.)

Germanium given by injection has helped people with chronic, degenerative diseases which are always immune related. Germanium is also available as capsules sold in health food stores.

Supplementation with these minerals will not cure candida, but they may provide necessary nutrients to the immune system.

Short-chain fatty acids

Fatty acids come in molecules of varying length. The short ones seem to work well in some people to inhibit candida growth. Caprylic (octanoic) acid, propionic acid, sorbic acid, and oleic acid are recommended to help fight candida. For this reason, olive oil (oleic acid) is often recommended and is easy to add to the diet. (Extra virgin olive oil should be used.)

These short-chain fatty acids work in much the same capacity as biotin in that they inhibit the conversion of yeast to its fungal form. Use of short-chain fatty acids does not destroy the beneficial bacteria, so it is a way to control candida while building up the beneficial bacteria colonies.

In addition to being a component of many foods, such as coconut, these simple fats are normally produced by beneficial bacteria in the G.I. tract. This by-product helps limit the growth of detrimental bacteria and fungi. When antibiotics kill much of the intestinal flora, the detrimental bacteria have a tendency to take over, particularly since most people eat a nutrient-depleted and fiber-deficient diet. This is how the problems with candidiasis and other fungal infections begins.

Therapy with short-chain fatty acids does not work for everyone and, when it does work, it takes about a month to notice improvements. And like the other therapies listed here, it does not cure candida, it only controls it by providing what should already be in the intestines were a proper bacteria culture present. But it can be an important step in relieving the symptoms of candida.

Such therapy means taking short-chain fatty acids in pill or tablet form as a dietary supplement. Tablets are usually coated to time-release further along in the G.I. tract so it is not absorbed too early and is available to inhibit candida where it is colonizing.

These supplements work in the G.I. tract and are not particularly effective for candida in the tissues. If candida involvement is limited to the G.I. tract, supplements like caprylic acid can work wonders, but will do only a little good for people with deep tissue candidiasis.

Linolenic and Linoleic Acids: (Evening Primrose Oil/ Flaxseed Oil / Black Currant Oil

During the last few years much as been written on the virtues of evening primrose oil (EPO). The research reports that EPO stimulates the immune system's T-Cells. Since candida attacks the T-cells, this may help. EPO provides gamma-linolenic acid used in many body functions as prostaglandins. The recommended dosage is 3-4000 mg. per day.

Black currant seed oil is even richer in gamma-linolenic acid than EPO, making it a new source of this factor.

Since EPO became popular, a lot of companies have jumped on the bandwagon to compete with each other. The products they offer are often inferior and the EPO is usually cut with other oils, vitamin E, and so forth. If you favor using EPO, use the pure oil, much of which comes from England.

Linseed oil is a rich source of linoleic acid, which also supports the immune system. But linseed oil is a by-product of the paint industry so it is of dubious quality. Fortunately, pure, cold-processed, refrigerated flaxseed oil in brown bottles is available and is probably the finest nutritinal oil in the world! [Look for Vegomega 3 by Spectrum in the refrigerator section of your health food store, or Systemic's FLX formula.

Flaxseed oil helps fight cholesterol, inhibits candida proliferation, and nourishes the entire body, especially the thyroid and nerves. This is covered in detail in the book *The Pro-Vita! Plan* along with instructions on how to make "balanced butter."

The reason these fatty acids come up when candida is a concern is that they're but another nutritional deficiency in most people — one that has a bearing on the immune system.

Vitamin C

Vitamin C is well-known for its support of the immune system — both as cleanser of toxins and as a nutrient to the T-cells — as well as for its support of individual cellular immunity. As a water soluble vitamin, vitamin C needs consistent replenishment, as it is lost from the body through the urine. If vitamin C is from a natural source and enzymated with herbs such as cinnamon and clove, it can be retained in the body as a nutrient instead of being flushed out as a cleanser. For candida, dosage varies with the individual. General recommendations are to keep the level at about 3000 mg/day or to let the body claim its own level, which is just below bowel intolerance — too much vitamin C causes diarrhea, drives copper out of the body, over-alkalizes (a reaction to the ascorbic acid), and can hemolize the red blood cells, making them die too quickly. Once again, proper dosage is important.

Perhaps we could stand a little honesty regarding vitamin C now that we've survived the scandal that revealed that much of the research on it was contrived — until the word finally got out.

The proper dosage of vitamin C varies with each individual. It's probably increasing due to the increasing amounts of pollutants in the air. But too much vitamin C can be detrimental, as already pointed out. Many of the articles on health would have us believe we can take bottles a day — the more the merrier. This is great for the vitamin companies, but not so great for the individual. Clinical anecdotal experience has shown that if two people coming down with colds take 10 grams of vitamin C, one forestalls the cold, the other gets it worse.

How vitamin C will react depends on the individual's biochemistry and pH balance. You cannot take a single, concentrated, isolated nutrient without affecting the whole body-system — sometimes it's beneficial, sometimes detrimental. Either use moderate amounts of low-potency, natural supplements, or consult with a professional clinical nutritionist.

Lactobacilli

Acidophilus and the other beneficial cultures (bifidus, thermophilus, Streptococcus faecium, bulgaricus) help balance the flora of the G.I. tract. Their effect is to crowd out yeast, ferment the sugars the yeast lives on, and excrete lactic acid, which inhibits yeast through the pH environment. Yeasts prefer an alkaline environment rather than acidic.

These beneficial "lac-bacs" produce nascent (ones newly created) B vitamins and natural antibiotics that serve to control disease-causing organisms with such infamous names as salmonella, streptococcus, E. coli, clostidium, diplococcus and staphylococcus. These detrimental organisms are known to synthesize cancer-causing compounds such as nitrosamines so the protection offered by the lac-bacs is quite important.

People are often led to believe that they can reinoculate the G.I. tract by taking acidophilus supplements or by adding yogurt or kefir to their diets. This doesn't seem to be the case, though supplementation with cultures does seem to help.

The doubt about the efficacy of taking these cultures is based on a couple of considerations. The first one is the difficulty in getting fully viable cultures. Some companies centrifuge their cultures, which separates the culture medium (usually milk) from the bacteria. This causes weak, nonviable cultures, but the product can be labeled and sold. Other cultures are old and many of the millions of bacteria claimed on the label are dead. Other companies sell cultures that are not normally found in the human G.I. tract. It only makes sense to use a strain found in humans and, of course, one that is known to be of reliable quality.

The other consideration is the ability of the culture to live on its journey through the stomach acid. It seems that once the first line of defense is established by the colostrum-based bacterial culture from the first nursings, the body then recognizes the G.I. tract as an invasion route, and, therefore, has evolved several systems to kill off any bacteria entering the tract thereafter. These first-line defenses include the hydrochloric acid in the stomach, the alkali of the duodenum, and the proper beneficial bacteria throughout the small and large intestine. With proper nutrition, the original culture was designed to last a lifetime. Acid-resistant strains have a greater chance of making it through the stomach and into the intestines. Time-release cultures offer a plan for inoculation in the small intestine.

Also, remember that a person's proper culture is unique — just as it was formed shortly after birth from the colostrum of the first few nursings — and it was intended to last a lifetime. Supplemental cultures do not approach the characteristics of the originally-established culture.

Many people's digestive systems are weakened by a lifetime of poor eating habits, such as improper food combinations, excessive animal proteins, and 20th-century stress. (A weakened digestive system is also a symptom of candida.) Because of this weakness some of the supplemental cultures do, indeed, pass through the stomach to live in the intestine, until they pass out of the body because they are unable to stick to the intestinal wall.

Having a digestive system weak enough to let acidophilus through also means it's weak enough to let viable yeast through. Food for thought.

To work effectively with acidophilus cultures in the G.I. tract, a good quality culture, fairly large quantity, and consistent use are the necessary factors.

One effective and inexpensive way to introduce "lac-bac" culture into the intestine is by drinking cabbage water or by eating raw sauerkraut. Cabbage teems with lac-bac. By soaking cabbage overnight in pure (non-chlorinated) water and drinking the water the next day, a high quality lac-bac can be introduced into the G.I. tract.

Raw sauerkraut, such as "Vegie Delight" is now available in the refrigerator section of health food stores. It is a wonderful, delicious, effervescent food teeming with beneficial culture.

There are other uses for acidophilus-type cultures. Rectal implants, IF they can be retained for several hours, can help balance the flora in the colon. Some nutritionists recommend such implants for people who've been fasting or taking colon irrigations (colonics) where the bowel is empty and the culture can be retained. But these implants cannot reach the small intestine due to the ileocecal valve, which blocks the way, so only part of the problem can be addressed in this way.

Acidophilus cultures make excellent douches, and can help normalize the flora in the vaginal area, thus helping to fight and prevent yeast infections. They also can help reduce the chance for, and retard the growth of, cancer cells.

There is a colostrum-based bifidus culture available in the U.S. now. It comes from Europe in both a lactose and non-dairy base. It has proven to be highly effective and offers the best approach to reseeding the G.I. tract available today. Japan has introduced a new bifidus in a food medium which is proving to be effective.

Potassium Permanganate

A couple more antifungal agents worth mentioning are from the chemistry set. Potassium permanganate is very strong and must be used with caution — externally only. In many places it's available only by prescription or from a chemical supply house that caters to chemists. 1/8 teaspoon to a bathtub of water is used to rid the skin of yeast and microscopic parasites. Soak for 15 minutes. Some people use this prior to close body contact with each other, to avoid exchanging fungus and yeast.

Potassium permanganate turns the water a deep burgundy color and can stain if more than 1/8 tsp. is used. But it is devastating to a wide variety of microorganisms that may inhabit the skin and genital area. In some drug stores it's sold over the counter, in others by prescription only.

Hydrogen Peroxide (H2O2)

Hydrogen peroxide (H2O2) is available over the counter. Bathing in a 1% solution accomplishes much the same as the bath in potassium permanganate, and it's safer in that the end product of hydrogen peroxide is water and oxygen. It is also an acid, so it supports proper skin pH. It can bleach clothing, so treat it as you would laundry bleach.

A therapy system has grown up around hydrogen peroxide. Its purported benefits are that it provides radical oxygen and that it kills bacteria, fungi and viruses. This therapy has been waxing and waning for over 40 years, but has never made a strong impression on the majority of health practitioners. More study is needed before anything conclusive can be presented. Such studies are now coming forth.

The reason that hydrogen peroxide therapy is so debatable is that it is based on incomplete viewpoints and on assumptions based on fragmented evidence — like so many other debatable issues. The basic issue is oxidants vs. antioxidants.

Elemental oxygen is known in chemistry to break molecules apart. It is an "oxidizer" or rust-promoting element. When oils oxidize they become rancid and quite poisonous. Skeptics of hydrogen peroxide therapy ask "why do you want to oxidize the body? Look at all the research on how anti-oxidants such as vitamin C, vitamin E, zinc, selenium promote health and protect us from oxidation and free radicals. By taking hydrogen peroxide, aren't you releasing free radicals known to cause cancer, aging, and disease?"

Proponents of hydrogen peroxide therapy reply that our bodies suffer due to lack of oxygen at the cellular level and contain far too many toxins because there's not enough oxygen to oxidize or burn up the toxins. The research of Dr. William Koch, some sixty years ago, showed that free radicals were the result of incomplete oxidation. Incomplete oxidation is caused by a lack of oxygen. The real issue seems to involve a question about the proper amount of oxygen. When combustion is optimal, the process does not cause aging and disease.

For an analogy, consider the automobile's combustion engine — if the mixture of fuel and air (oxygen) is too rich or too lean, combustion is poor and the by-products cause greater pollution than a properly tuned engine. The same is true of human beings, but we're talking about combustion at the cellular level. Not enough oxygen results in free-radicals, toxins, fermentations — all synonymous with disease. Too much oxygen (if it were possible), would result in the burning of the tissues.

Deadly free radicals can be released by oxygen-releasing free radicals from chemical toxins in the body. Let's not make the mistake of blaming the oxygen. Let's look at the poisons we buy at the supermarket — vegetables sprayed with insecticides, meat loaded with antibiotics and steroids, hydrogenated oils, chemical preservatives and additives.

There is just cause for concern regarding the depletion of the Earth's oxygen-creating jungles and forests and the effects of air

108

pollution that reduces the amount of planetary oxygen. In addition, many medical drugs deplete oxygen from the body. Ordinary asprin interferes with the hemoglobin's ability to carry oxygen. It's possible to say that taking an aspirin a day for the heart contributes to cancer in some other organ if we view cancer as an anerobic (lack of oxygen) disease.

Getting more oxygen into our bloodstream is a basic, vital concern. Nobel prize-winning doctor, Otto Warburg, showed that most cancers occur in an anaerobic environment — one lacking oxygen. In a state of oxygen deprivation, cells turn to fermentation for energy, which leads to autointoxication (self poisoning) and to abnormal behaviors such as forming tumors and cancers. It is widely accepted that many forms of cancer are cellular fermentations. Death results from autointoxication (starvation) rather than the disease.

From a nutritional perspective, oxygen is the breath of life. An oxygen-rich bloodstream brings sparkling vitality, stamina, and freedom from infections and most diseases. Note: We're saying most diseases because new varieties of aerobic cancers — ones that can survive in the presence of oxygen — have been found, thus stimulating new research efforts.

A variety of tests are being conducted now on the uses of H2O2, including the use of food grade (35%) hydrogen peroxide diluted in distilled water and drunk as a therapy, as well as the injection of .05% hydrogen peroxide intravenously. Results are well-documented showing a reduction of bacteria, virus, and parasites. So are side effects (nausea, heavy detoxification reactions, hemolized red blood cells, and kidney stress).

In laboratory rats, tumors in the small intestine were found when H2O2 was given orally. It seems that as long as the peroxide enters the bloodstream through the stomach or intravenously there is no problem with G.I. tract tumors. Such tumors may have been caused by a reaction with other elements. Some damage has been done by rectal implants of H2O2 when it wasn't diluted enough.

When proper research is completed, hydrogen peroxide research may provide answers to many health problems. Some people have overcome infections and toxemia through its use. Actually oxygen will prove to be the healer. It remains to be seen what the best source of oxygen is.

Researchers against the internal use of hydrogen peroxide cite these arguments:

Hydrogen peroxide

- is released by the body under certain conditions and for highly specific reasons; it is not for general use.

- kills both good and bad bacteria, and like an antibiotic,   it damages the body in the process of ridding it of microorganisms, thus candida returns when the H2O2 therapy ends.

- contributes to aging through the production of hydroxyl radicals.

- inhibits brain enzymes.

- inhibits the normal activity of sympathetic nerve fiber.

- inhibits the immune system (inhibits immunoglobulin).

- causes cellular damage (Heinz bodies).

- damages the eyes (lipid peroxidation in the lens).

- injures the duodenum (gastric erosion).

- damages cartilage.

- causes heart damage (toxic derivatives).

- interferes with nerve function.

- may cause genetic damage (breaks in DNA chains).

- increases the rate of mercury vapor uptake in the blood.

- causes red blood cells to stiffen thus they are less able to bend and flow in capilaries.

Keep in mind that H2O2 advocates have answers for many of these claims. The different opinions clash and, for the time being, people must decide for themselves.

The wisdom of experience would tell us that, in the health arena when opposing views are so adamant, it is usually a case of neither side being 100% right and neither case being 100% wrong.

The case for increasing the intake of oxygen is well-founded. Whether or not hydrogen peroxide is the most appropriate tool for increasing that intake remains to be seen. Many people opt for the

STABILIZED oxygens, to avoid the potential dangers of hydrogen peroxide, while still obtaining the benefits of increased oxygen.

A recent beneficial use of H2O2 comes from Europe where they put it in milk. Once treated this way, the milk stays fresh for months without refrigeration. At a time when the U.S. government is trying to sell us on the idea of irradiating our food with gamma radiation from nuclear wastes, H2O2 may be a viable alternative to the devastating effects of radiation on the quality and life-force of our food.

In our clinical tests, doctor-injected H2O2 provided the most dramatic results, clearing the blood of rod form bacteria, fungi, and tubules. However, within 2-3 weeks, after discontinuing the injections, the microorganisms reappeared. From this we conclude that H2O2 injections-helped, but only provided temporary results. Furthermore, we observed oxidative damage to the red blood cells, verifying the concern that H2O2 damages tissue.

Oral ingestion of H2O2 showed much slower response, and large doses were required to cause a change in the blood — dosages often resulting in nausea and cleansing reactions. There are a number of potential dangers in drinking H2O2. Should the H2O2 act on fats, they will release rancid elements known to cause cancer. Reactions with certain salts, such as iron salts, can create toxic side effects. Normally H2O2 is absorbed through the stomach without problems, but should it enter the small intestine the probability of toxic reaction is greatly increased. This is simply the natural function of the oxygen radical (O1) — to oxidize toxins so they can be eliminated. The problem is not with the oxygen, but with our highly toxic bodies. At some time and by some method, we must detoxify.

The proper use of H2O2 is a debatable issue. Here's one use that even the H2O2 advocates have yet to discover. It is a helpful therapy for subcutaneous candida infestation.

Mix 1/4 cup H2O2 (3%) with 1/4 cup baking soda (NaOH). This combination makes a sodium oxide that is many times more effective at killing fungus than the H2O2 alone. Plus, the carbonic acid in this mixture allows the free oxygen radical easier access to the cells. It serves as a cell penetrant. The alkaline baking soda buffers the caustic action making the H2O2 safer as well as more effective. This is a therapy for occasional, temporary use.

The baking soda/H2O2 mixture can be used occasionally (once or twice a month) as a body scrub, (avoid contact with the hair, unless you are willing to risk the hair-lightening, color changing effects), mouth wash, toothpaste, and antifungal for fungus under the toenails. Note: If you have dandruff, you have candida on the scalp. This mixture will also lighten liver (age) spots. For hair, the natural, antifungal shampoo (Fanie White Oak Shampoo) mentioned in "Subcutaneous Candida Incubation" is best. For daily use, the Fanie Sweet Birch body cleanser is an excellent skin cleanser with antifungal properties. [Fanie products are based on the research of Dr. Clyde Johnson.]

It's worth a mention here that there is no such thing as a panacea — a miracle cure for all people. What works for one person does not necessarily work for another. Different metabolic orientations (anabolic/catabolic) react differently to H2O2 therapy, so in some situations H2O2 may help, in others it will hurt.

This is not mentioned by the H2O2 proponents who may not be familiar with Dr. Emmanuel Revici's work on the subject. Some proponents of H2O2 therapy are also engaged in selling hydrogen peroxide at premium prices. In Texas, 35% food grade hydrogen peroxide is readily available at $7.00/gallon wholesale, and the price is drastically reduced for 55 gallon quantities. Proponents sell it for $16.00/pint, or $128.00/gallon in the wake of all the panacea claims.

It remains to be seen if hydrogen peroxide is a viable way to add oxygen to our hypoxic (under-oxygenated) bodies, but many people testify to its temporary benefits. Nature's cleanser, anti-infective, and energizer is oxygen. It's role is to enliven and purify. The O1 radical derived from hydrogen peroxide is highly reactive and shows great promise in controlling candida in the blood, but at what cost?

A company in Dallas makes a stabilized elemental oxygen that they claim is more effective than H2O2 and much safer. It's certainly worth looking into. Instead of a radical oxidation, it provides oxygen that can be retained and used more discriminately by the body. It also keeps bacteria out of the water cooler and does not alter the taste of the water like hydrogen peroxide does. Also, in 1987, a California-based company began marketing stabilized oxygen.

We add stabilized oxygen to our home-made baby formula, drinking water, and any open jar for longer shelf life.

There is no doubt about the beneficial qualities of oxygen. It remains to be seen, in the midst of the H2O2 craze, if hydrogen peroxide is the best way to obtain the oxygen. For now, oxygen (particularly stabilized oxygen) helps and that makes it a valuable ally in fighting candida, fungus, and other infections.

EMOTIONS AS CAUSE AND CURE

In the late 1970s, the importance of emotional states as a cause and cure of disease came to the forefront of the natural health movement. In the book *Energy and Addictions* the health triad is presented portraying the importance of attitude in a person's level of health.

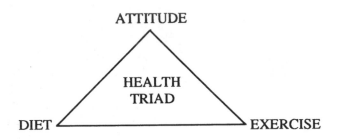

No healing system is complete unless it addresses the underlying emotional states (energy patterns) and offers methods for healing at that level.

I asked Austin health counselor Jessie Keener-Clark, N.D., to present her insights on candida as she has direct experience in helping people with Candidiasis with her "Integrative Breathing" technique. According to her:

"The connection between candida-related disorders and our emotions is subtle and underlying, yet the implications are profound. In explaining this relationship it may be useful to review a physical quality of Candidiasis, which is that the yeast fungus is proliferating **out of control** in the body. The immune system is unable to control the fungus, and the symptoms produced can be equally unmanageable."

"Research has shown that before the body physically manifests disease, the energy of that disease is present. All disease begins on an energetic level. What then is the energy that allows Candidiasis to manifest?"

"Emotional patterning, thoughts, and feelings all produce energetic reactions in the physical body. The outstanding "pattern" that candida patients have in common, in my experience, is that they prefer to be in control of themselves, their lives, situations, and circumstances. At first glance this appears to be a normal, acceptable desire in civilized humans. After all, who wants to lose control of the way society views them, or of the car they're driving, or their bodily functions? In fact, not being in control is a very scary prospect to most people!"

"But let's look at this from a deeper perspective: What we're attempting to control is life-force energy — thoughts, ideas, and feelings, which then are projected into actions and reactions. The basic premise is that we're safe, as long as we're in control. Such an attitude is self-limiting because life is not always controllable. In fact, one reality we know to be true in our lives is that everything changes. We can't always control the outcome, or even the process of change. The key is not whether we can or cannot control, but how we respond when we're not in control. We feel unsafe! This is the very energy that Candida albicans fungus feeds on. What the fungus (which reproduces out of control) seems to thrive on is our fear of being out of control. This has been illustrated quite clearly using bio-kinesiology techniques."

"Using affirmations, or positive statements, is an effective way to change the emotional energy that can promote candida growth. The intention is to create a feeling of safety, regardless of the control status. A helpful affirmation would be: "I am absolutely safe, whether I am in control or not." This particular statement may seem innocuous at first, but I've had clients burst into tears (or peals of laughter) upon hearing it. One client responded, through her sobs, 'But I'm not safe, I'm not!'"

"Clearly her fear of not being in control was a driving force in her life, and motivated her to always be in control or, in other words, she was operating out of fear. (Much research has been done linking fear with disease processes.) By repeating this affirmation often, she created a new feeling of certainty in her life. Her candida symptoms (constipation and P.M.S.) were greatly reduced in her first month of following nutritional programs and weekly counseling sessions. The big difference, however, was in her personal life. She reported an increasing sense of well-being.

Her finances and relationships improved. She even learned to use her affirmation as an immediate response to stress, and found it particularly helpful in coping with being stuck in traffic jams."

"The effectiveness of this type of therapy is directly proportional to the client's willingness to change. An affirmation is worthless if it is not used, and the more it is used (repeated out loud or written), the more quickly the physical body integrates the energy of that thought. Often it is appropriate for person to do "Integrative Breathing" (a self-help technique involving connected breathing and repeated affirmations) to integrate their fears more quickly."

"This new energy will change the vibrational energy of the physical body to the point of preventing or changing a disease process. Such an approach to disease has been documented by many leading healers and health practitioners, including John Diamond, M.D., and Louise Hay."

"Candida is not the cause. It is a symptom. Emotionally, the cause is a great fear, common to us all, of not being in control. By integrating this fear (becoming one with it, so that it's no longer something to be resisted), we change our vibratory rate to one that is no longer suitable for candida proliferation."

Some additional affirmations for candida are:

1. The Universe is a safe place for me to be.

2. I give up my fear of healing completely.

3. I am no longer afraid of fear. It keeps me safe by warning me of danger or by changing my negative thoughts.

4. My negative patterns are now dissolving effortlessly.

5. I am no longer a helpless victim. I love taking responsibility for my creativity."

VAGINAL CONSIDERATIONS

Let's look at some of the ways yeast can be introduced into or yeast-proliferation can occur within the vagina, in particular.

Sexual activity: Candida can be classified as a venereal disease since it can be transmitted either way, from or to either partner, by sexual activity.

Antibiotics: For whatever reason they are used, they kill the lactobacillus in the vaginal area, as well as in the G.I. tract, upsetting the flora in the vaginal area and weakening its natural defenses.

Menstrual period: Candida prefers an alkaline environment, and during menstruation the vagina becomes alkaline, primarily because the pH of the blood is 7.2-7.4 (alkaline). Vaginal pH is normally around 4.5 (acid).

Birth control pills: The female hormone, progesterone, is a component of birth control pills. It is known to encourage candida proliferation by its action of preparing glycogen for use as sugar for cellular energy. Some researchers think this gives candida-fungus a food source at the cellular level. This also accounts for the typical postmenstrual yeast infection, since the natural progesterone hormone levels are higher after ovulation and blood is an excellent medium for growing candida cultures a few days later.

Improper wiping: This causes a variety of vaginal complaints, as there are numerous infectious bacteria in the colon. Wiping from back to front exposes the vaginal area to the candida and fungi from the colon. Wiping from front to back helps avoid this contamination.

Tampons: This may not be such an issue since the public is aware of the toxic shock syndrome. Keeping a foreign object that may have airborne yeast on it in a warm, moist, alkaline environment provides ideal circumstances for culturing yeast, as does retaining the blood for long periods of time. Changing tampons frequently seems to be the rule now to avoid problems.

Feminine hygiene sprays: These sprays often provide irritants that cause immune reactions, altered pH, and indirectly contribute to candida and vaginitis.

Synthetic undergarments: These can cause excessive sweating, particularly in warm climates, which provides the moist environment required by candida. Air needs to circulate around the body. Cotton undergarments allow circulation. The synthetics, such as nylon and polyester, prevent proper circulation.

Maintaining an acid pH is important to vaginal health. If the pH becomes alkaline, douching with acidophilus, or hydroxyquinoline sulfate (1 tbsp./pint — an extract of grapefruit rind often used topically for complexion and fungal problems) will help acidify the vaginal area and thus prevent candida proliferation. Apple cider vinegar is not recommended since it contains live yeasts.

RELATED CONSIDERATIONS AND INTERLINKED SYMPTOMS

Several areas of health can be closely connected to Candidiasis or completely independent. Yet if they are connected to candida, there will be no lasting improvement until candida is brought under control, preferably eliminated.

These areas of interlinked, interrelated symptoms include hypoglycemia, food allergies, obesity, and premenstrual syndrome (PMS).

We'll briefly take a look at these complications and how they relate to Candidiasis.

HYPOGLYCEMIA

Candidiasis is a major cause of hypoglycemia (low blood sugar) and hypoglycemic symptoms occur because the candida interferes with the enzymes responsible for sugar metabolism. Also, the additional burden that Candidiasis puts on the liver and the adrenal glands means that candida interferes with the whole blood sugar maintenance process.

Hypoglycemia is a condition where the blood sugar levels drop too low producing symptoms such as fatigue, depression, fuzzy-thinking, extreme hunger and sugar cravings, and muscle weakness.

The blood sugar levels drop due to an inability of the body to regulate its blood sugar system properly.

Let's first look at the basic process for an understanding of hypoglycemia. Although various forms of hypoglycemia exist and can often be suspected when people display a strong hunger and irritability just before meal time, hypoglycemia as a disease label only exists when three criteria are met:

1. The blood glucose level must be well under the normal range as determined by a blood test,

2. The patient's symptoms must only occur when blood glucose levels are too low,

3. The patient's symptoms must disappear when simple sugars are eaten.

What we're investigating is the body's supply of its basic metabolic fuel - glucose. Is the fuel readily and consistently available, or is it sometimes too high, too low, or unavailable?

The body has a system whereby it maintains its supply of fuel (glucose) and makes it available to the cells via insulin.

' Four organs are interrelated in blood sugar and form a team for the proper maintenance of energy for the body. The thyroid pancreas, the adrenals, and the liver. Nutritionally speaking, these three organs/glands must be supported for succcess in a hypoglycemia program, yet unfortunately most programs only focus on the pancreas and thus experience only temporary success.

One aspect of diet is the foods eaten become fuel for the body. Note: This is only one aspect of food. People often make the mistake of viewing food solely as materials for energy. Food is much more than materials for energy. It must also provide the building blocks of tissue, the enzymes for thousands of chemical reactions, and the raw materials (minerals, oils, amino acids, vitamins) for countless molecular functions. Energy is only a small role of diet.

The energy system is very simple. Carbohydrates are broken down into sugars, converted into glucose for cellular energy, and a supply of this fuel is maintained by the body.

The energy system was designed to function optimally on complex carbohydrates which are gradually broken down into glucose for energy. Refined sugars rush the normal process causing the sugar regulating system to be stressed.

So the eating of refined sugars, sodas, candies, ice cream, pastries, etc. is the first stress which leads to hypoglycemia. It ususally takes a few years to develop. Hypoglycemia was one of the first symptoms of the junk food era — one where people's diets became too rich in refined sugars and too low in nutrients (vitamins, minerals, etc.)

One of several functions of the pancreas is to produce the hormone insulin. On anticipating a food supply, the pancreas produces insulin which serves as an escort system for glucose to enter the cells. When blood sugar rises, insulin moves it into the cells thus helping to maintain a fairly constant level in the blood.

The liver converts the simple sugars into glucose for the body to have its preferred fuel supply. Therefore, it is up to the liver to make the proper fuel. The proper fuel for a combustion engine Ford or Chevy is gasoline, not jet fuel, not diesel. The liver constructs the proper fuel for the body which is glucose in a proper matrix of amino acids, fatty acids, and minerals which are also in serum. The thyroid regulates the pace of liver function.

The liver has the ability to store glucose in the form of glycogen, a super-concentrated packet of energy, for use later should the need arise. The liver can also convert amino acids (proteins) and fats into glucose should the need arise.

So the body has a system in place to provide the basic fuel for its cells and guarantee a supply of fuel under many adverse circumstances should they occur — times of abundance (poor combinations of foods), times of famine, times of imbalance (lack of carbohydrates).

When we understand the importance of the liver and how much responsibility it has to regulate blood sugar, we soon realize that hypoglycemia is much more a liver problem than it is a pancreas problem.

The adrenal glands are also involved in the blood sugar loop. They produce hormones to counteract insulin in the event too much is produced. Also, should blood sugar levels drop too low, a potentially life threatening occurance, the adrenal glands secrete hormones (glucagon, adrenalin, norepinephrine, cortisol, etc.) to stabilize blood sugar. This is an "above and beyond the call of duty" job for the adrenals, but they are often called upon to perform this duty by people who eat refined sugars (sweets).

The hormonal rush from the adrenal glands is basically a fight or flight response, and not supposed to be an everyday occurance. Side effects of using the adrenal system are anger, anxiety, dizziness, excessive perspiration, fears, heart palpitations, irritability, restlessness of limbs, shakiness, etc. [For more information on the thyroid and adrenals, see: *The Next Step To Greater Energy.*]

So, now that we're familiar with the body systems and backup systems regarding the maintenance of blood sugar, let's look at how the system breaks down.

Hypoglycemia is caused by several conditions including nutrient deficiency, overweight, and sedentary lifestyle, but the major cause is the overeating of refined sugars. Since it is well documented that eating refined sugars contributes to nutrient deficiency and obesity, it's the candies and soda pop that emerge as the primary cause.

Some researchers think that the smallpox vaccination can damage the pancreas and establish the potential for hypoglycemia or the other side of the blood sugar coin, diabetes, to occur.

When a person eats highly concentrated sugars, the pancreas gets the message to produce a lot of insulin, which it does. The inrush of sugar stresses the liver to produce glucose and the insulin, now in abundance in the blood, carries the glucose into the cells. As it works out, too much insulin is produced so the adrenals may need to get into the act to try to counteract the excessive insulin. The end result is the blood sugar ends in a deficit and the blood sugar maintenance system has been overworked.

When this occurs day after day, the blood sugar regulatory system becomes stressed, less able to perform its tasks. Hypoglycemia becomes established as the best the body can do with what it has to work with. If the hypoglycemia continues, it's only a matter of time until there is further breakdown of the pancreas and diabetes results.

Also, people who rely on sweets frequently can warp their body's ability read what the diet is providing. When complex carbohydrates are eaten the body does not recognize them as a sugar (when compared to ice cream) and thus insulin is not produced resulting in altered metabolism and low blood sugar. Once the system is stressed there are a number of ways it can fall apart.

A system under stress is prey to candida involvement. Usually the stressed body gets a bacterial infection somewhere and an antibiotic is given paving the way for candida proliferation.

Candida also likes the environment of fluctuating blood sugar levels (the high sugars give candida a boost) and the hormonal emergency system provides both food and an immune-suppressive condition favorable to candida.

Once candida is established, there will be little success in treating the hypoglycemia until the candida is taken care of. Such people need to go on a full candida program augmented by liver, adrenal, and pancreas support.

This is so common, that the comprehensive candida program presented in this material automatically includes a phase of working with the pancreas. The "Liver Triad Program" should always follow the candida program.

Hypoglycemia is diagnosed via a glucose tolerance test which requires six hours to complete. During the test, people are often given a glucose syrup to drink which is made from corn. If a person has a corn allergy, the blood sugar will drop as part of their allergic reaction and hypoglycemia will be misdiagnosed.

In addition to the six hour glucose tolerance test, there are other ways to susect if you are involved with a hypoglycemic reaction. One is questionnaires provided by your health professional. In Sclerology, if there are stress lines affecting the pancreas, adrenals, and liver, we always suspect blood sugar regulatory difficulties.

From the natural healing perspective, it is not important to diagnose hypoglycemia. Knowing the sugar regulatory system is stressed, regardless what it is called (as long as glucose is not passing in the urine), is enough, and proper nutritional therapy and diet can begin.

In the old days when hypoglycemia was in vogue, doctors would recommend a high protein diet. While this temproarily allayed the symptoms, it was detrimental to the whole person's health. (The high proteins caused acidosis, taxed the liver, depleted calcuim and sodium, and stressed the adrenals.) Now, a diet centered around complex carbohydrates is recommended and this works much better. Optimally, a person could go on the Pro-Vita! Plan using complex carbohydrates for lunch and supper, and for snacks if needed to maintain blood sugar and keep the body off the roller coaster of reactions to sugar. The optimal protein matrix of the Pro-Vita! diet helps rebuild the overtaxed organs/glands so the body can rebuild and recover.

CANDIDA AND FOOD ALLERGIES

We've already discussed how candida can cause food allergies and food allergies can cause candida. For people involved in both concerns, a dual program should be undertaken. It's a difficult pathway, one which may take a year to stabilize, but the sooner started, the sooner relief will appear.

People involved in both allergies and candida are often environmentally sensitive and require comprehensive nutritional support, careful administration of natural therapies, and a host of attributes such as patience, perseverance, dedication, etc.

Work with such conditions may involve avoidance of allergenic foods, nutritional support to help break food addictions (addictions are often based on allergies), homeopathic potentizations of food allergins, nosodes for Epstein Barr (often associated with allergies), short fasts, full candida programs, clearing of free radicals from the diet and body, homeopathic phenolic neutralizations, and supplements to build the endocrine, hepatic, and immune system.

With a carefully monitored program, each phase of the program can build on the previous success and the patient can become stable quickly, and then begin the more lengthy program of rebuilding.

The allergy/candida patients require the assistance of a dedicated health professional.

Obesity and Candidiasis

Both Candidiasis and food allergies can contribute to obesity. There are several other factors also involved such as the appestat center, metabolic rate, caloric (sugar) intake, level of stress, the "fat thermostat", the need for nurture, lack of exercise, and so forth.

Candida is involved with obesity in many ways. So the removal of candidiasis can automatically help people lose the excessive weight. Candida should be investigated as a contributing factor in obesity in every instance.

Here are nine ways Candidiasis causes obesity.

1. One of the responses of the body to toxins whether they be chemical, environmental, dietary, a result of candida, or a result of antigenic food particles, is to surround the toxin with fat and store it in the adipose tissues. The body may also surround the toxin with water. If the liver is unable to process the toxins and release them to the kidneys (they may be unable to process the water), the toxins build up as fat and water retentiveness, both of which contribute to excessive weight.

2. Since Candidiasis causes fatigue, sufferers are reluctant to exercise and the muscles have a short supply of nutrient availability due to candida's interference in the system. A lack of exercise is known contributor to obesity. And on the positive side, exercise raises the metabolic rate causing the burning of fat.

3. Candidiasis interferes with the thyroid hormone function. The thyroid gland may be doing its job just fine producing thyroxin and other hormones, but candida interferes with the body's utilization of hormones resulting in the normal blood test scores (T-3, T-4, T-7) but all the symptoms of low thyroid such as cold hands and feet. Since the thyroid hormones regulate the body's thermostat or rate energy is combusted, an impaired combustion rate results in excess cellular energy which becomes stored as fat.

4. The body has the ability to maintain its weight by creating energy (to a certain extent) and by wasting energy at the cellular level so excesses can be used up. The hormones produced as a result of stress and the stress of Candidiasis on the system can impair the body's ability to use up excessive cellular energy. This results in a storage of the excessive energy as fat. Diets that push the limit of the energy wasting system (refined carbohydrates) readily contribute to obesity when the system is impaired.

5. Candidiasis tricks the body into believing it is running low on energy and nutrients. The hormones which appear to help the body deal with the stress of candida can make the hypothalmus interpret the situation as starvation. The hypothalmus then keeps the hunger button pushed so the person will eat to provide energy and nutrients. The excessive hunger causes excessive eating. A person then may start to skip breakfast (a big mistake) to lower the total amount of food eaten. This is interpreted by the hypothalmus

as a starvation situation and it will set the metabolic rate to a "store fat, times are lean" mode. And thus the person eats less and gains more weight. Until candida is addressed, the person will live a dieter's hell experiencing failure with every attempt.

6. Candidiasis causes excessive hunger and a craving for carbohydrate and sugar-based foods. The yeast toxins interfere with the very enzyme systems which are responsible for providing fuel to the cells. The foods that appear to satisfy this are the sugars and this leads to the hypoglycemic reaction. Food addictions are also involved in the same process. But the bottom line is the person is hungry, eats a lot, the body stores the calories as fat, and thus obesity results.

7. Candidiasis impairs the metabolism of fats, so obese people have trouble getting rid of fat if they have Candidiasis. Fat is normally burned in the muscles and obese people are often deficient in exercise. And even if an exercise program were undertaken, candida interferes with the very process of burning fat by impairing the beta-oxidation enzymes required for that specific process. The eating of sweets raises insulin levels which in turn cause the body to store fats. Once stored, fats must be split by an enzyme into fatty acids and glycerol which can then be utilized for energy or burned up. Toxins from candida interfere with these basic processes resulting in an inability to burn the fat.

8. Candidiasis impairs the metabolism of sugars causing a breakdown in a person's metabolic system and a reliance on carbohydrates in the diet to provide quick energy since the body's metabolic system is not functioning well. This contributes to the excessive use of carbohydrates and the storage of calories as fat.

9. Candidiasis impairs the introduction of glucose into the cells because of its toxins which cause the release of stress hormones. If the body reads this as too much glucose in the blood and not in the cells, it will secrete more insulin to deal with the apparent excessive glucose. Insulin, in addition to helping the glucose move into the cells, also tells the body to store glucose as fat. Excessive amounts also inhibit fat metabolism. So, candida puts the body into a higher than needed insulin state and the body's reaction is to add fat.

Now you can see how so many weight loss programs simply fight themselves and why there are so many failures. It's like pushing in on a door that opens outward.

The basic point here is Candidiasis makes a mess out of the basic life support systems of the body, its utilization of nutrients and metabolic processes. Eliminating candida and correcting the cause is a fundamental step to restore health.

The body has fabulous systems in place to run its day to day operations. Only by returning to a lifestyle in accord with natural law can we hope to have optimal health. Most people's 20th-century lifestyles have created the need for 20th-century drugs (antibiotics), which have created the disease candidiasis, which is disrupting the very foundation of human health. It's not all medicine's fault.

What we need is to develop a basic understanding of ourselves as whole beings — chemistry, energy, emotions, thoughts, soul — in relation to the life force that animates our experiences. Nature does not forgive ignorance. It is up to each of us to educate ourselves and learn the principles to live by. That's probably why you are reading this now.

Premenstrual Syndrome and Candidiasis

PMS and Candidiasis are closely related since the female hormonal system is another system which operates within a delicate balance - one which candida has a proclivity to unbalance, and both are associated with carbohydrate metabolism, and hormonal function.

Simply put, if you have candida, and if you are a woman prior to menopause, you most likely will have symptoms of PMS.

The following symptoms are common amoung PMS sufferers: bloating, headaches, breast swelling and tenderness, light and noise sensitivity, acne, rashes, herpes outbreaks before periods, leg cramps, accident-proneness, hunger, sinusitis, ovarian pain (one sided), joint pain, backache, sugar cravings, and alcohol sensitivity.

PMS is noted for mood symptoms which include: anger, fear, restlessness, paranoia, inability to cope, forgetfulness, inability to concentrate, insecurity, change in sex drive, self-blame, sadness, depression, mental fatigue, guilt, irritability, and loneliness.

To understand why so much is at stake, let's first look at the menstrual cycle from a hormonal viewpoint.

Day one of the menstrual cycle is the day that the period starts. The average cycle lasts 28 days and starts again with the onset of menstrual bleeding. Ovulation (releasing the egg from the ovary) usually occurs around the 14th day of the cycle.

At ovulation, the progesterone hormone begins to increase in the blood and stays high until around day 24 when it rapidly decreases and is virtually gone at the onset of the next cycle.

PMS symptoms occur or worsen when progesterone is high prior to the period and cease or lessen considerably when progesterone is low or absent.

The cause of the PMS symptoms is not really well defined, but several theories make a great deal of sense and most of them relate directly to Candidiasis.

Candida feeds on progesterone. With yeast being a normal inhabitant of our planet, and women's progesterone levels naturally increasing as part of their menstrual cycle, the potential for yeast involvement is ever present. To a healthy body, the increase of yeast is something that is well maintained. To a body that cannot cope with the additional stress, candida can flare up in the presence of progesterone and contribute to the PMS symptoms.

Once again, candida-related PMS is simply a symptom that the immune system is under stress and is not coping fully with its challenges.

The toxins produced by the increased amount of candida can interfere with the cellular absorption of progesterone as well as other hormones. Hormones cannot perform their function unless they are introduced into the cell. This results in a high level of progesterone in the blood that cannot get into the cells. This quite likely results in an imbalance between progesterone and estrogen or an estrogen reaction to too much progesterone and thus the various symptoms occur due to the hormonal imbalance.

Candida metabolism produces toxins, some of which closely resemble estrogen. We mentioned that brewers yeast as a dietary supplement could contain estrogens and estrogen-precursers, and the same is true of living yeasts in the body. If the body is harboring high amounts of candida, the estrogen-like production of its metabolic wastes can be enough to create a hormonal imbalance.

Furthermore, the toxic metabolic wastes of candida can bind with estrogen or inhibit estrogens receptivity by cells resulting in a lack of estrogen in the cells and too much in the blood.

So to keep it simple, and as we've learned so far, candida messes up the not only the metabolic system but the hormonal system as well.

Both of these are serious effects of a simple micro-organism gone unchecked in the body.

DIET

Brace yourself! You may not have to follow the traditional, restrictive candida diets to be successful in conquering candida — at least not to the extent preached in the popular books. And then again, such a diet may be quite necessary. All the other candida diet books fail to provide the criteria for determining this.

In our clinical research we have found that people often over-restrict themselves and fail because the diet was too stringent. Following a diet requires a little information and a little finesse. Also, the quality of the supplementation program has a great bearing on the ability to succeed at a diet.

One of the things commonly associated with candidiasis is the so-called candida diet. Many people dread finding out they have yeast/fungus involvement more because of the restrictive diet so many authorities promote than because of the disease itself.

Restrictive diets are a double-edged sword: They can help and they can hurt.

From the health food consumer's perspective, one of the difficult aspects of a candida diet is that some of the all-time favorite health foods now become enemies — molds on alfalfa sprouts, whole wheat bread, fruit, mushrooms (fungi), apple cider vinegar, etc. [Note: Don't give up the sprouts. Soak them in the Chlorox or H2O2 bath to rid them of molds as outlined in *The Pro Vita! Plan* and at the end of this book.

The primary reason for restricting the diet by eliminating everything that feeds yeasts is simply to cut off the yeasts' food source so proliferation is limited. This is an attempt to starve it out. It is also an attempt to prevent additional viable yeasts from entering the G.I. tract.

The reasons diet restrictions can hurt are as follows: 1) Since candida proliferation occurs in a nutrient-depleted environment, further restriction of diet can make it even harder to get needed nutrients. It is quite common for people with candidiasis to exhibit a number of nutritional deficiencies, particularly of biotin and other B vitamins, zinc, germanium, vitamins A and E, and available amino acids.

2) Another reason is more philosophical but, nevertheless, quite valid. Restriction begets restriction. Once foods are eliminated, the body will find something in whatever is left in the diet to become sensitive to. Once that is eliminated, the body will find something else in what's still being eaten. This can continue until there are only one or two foods that can be tolerated. And since these aren't being rotated, they too can become allergins. This has really happened. Check it out with environmentally sensitive people who've not made a conscientious effort to add foods to their diet. The list of safe foods gets smaller and smaller.

The trick with candidiasis is to restrict only those foods that definitely cause a reaction. This nearly always includes a few items such as beer, bread, wine, mushrooms, apple cider vinegar, and all sugars. Many other items must be decided case by case, as we'll see.

Wheat bread, for example, may need to be eliminated, but corn bread may not. Sourdough bread may cause flare-ups, but an occasional piece of pita bread may not. It all depends on what aggravates the candida and how effective the nutritional therapy is.

We need a clear perspective on diet, because it is NOT the primary cause of yeast in the human body. Remember we talked about yeast filling the air? Every breath you take draws yeast into the body. If your immune system is already weakened, airborne yeasts are a major offender.

People interested in restricting yeast might do better to restrict breathing. Since this is not practical, everyone picks on diet. If a nutritional program is truly effective, many of the little diet restrictions that create such stress due to failed attempts will not be necessary. These restrictions will not have as much impact as a nutritional program that is strong enough to overcome the airborne yeasts and the already-established internal yeasts.

Subcutaneous yeast incubation may be a much larger problem than G.I. tract infection. Evaluation by a trained nutritionist can lead to the proper approach.

The major food offenders for people with Candidiasis include; bread, fruit and fruit juice, apple cider vinegar, mushrooms, beer, wine, sugars (sweets), and alfalfa sprouts (unless treated to rid them of mold). These offenders should be eliminated until candida is conquered, which includes a strong immune system and a healthy flora in the G.I. tract. Even then, persistent use of these items and continued stress may contribute to candida's return.

Many candida diets eliminate fermented foods such as miso, tofu, vinegar, tempeh, and rejuvalac (a fermented wheat berry drink), which sounds like a good idea until advocates of the macrobiotic diet report that one of the misos (fermented soy bean paste) can inhibit yeast. Rejuvalac is full of yeasts, except when it can be fermented with only lactobacillus, and that will then make it a yeast fighter.

Many candida diets suggest that you eliminate cheese because of the molds and yeasts it contains. This sounded reasonable until some people experienced anti-candida results from taking French Roquefort cheese with pineapple juice. This was an effort to inoculate the G.I. tract with the penicillin-type bacteria in the cheese that would kill off some of the yeast. This is particulary useful to people in the critical, "level 4," stage when the stomach burns or hurts so much they can't take pills. After a few treatments with one ounce of French Roquefort along with six ounces of pineapple juice, they are then able to use supplements. Also, French feta cheese in moderation does not seem to promote yeasts. (The Greeks use many pesticides and chemicals around the sheep, goats, and cows whose milk makes cheese, whereas in France this is prohibited. The French feta is preferable to the Greek for that reason.) As you can see, there are exceptions to many of the rules laid down by candida diet proponents.

Vinegar is another exception. Many people react violently to raw apple cider vinegar when they have candidiasis. Some people are helped by other vinegars, as they acidify, and thus restrict the yeast's environment, as well as promote digestion. Different vinegars have different effects on yeast. The two least offensive natural vinegars are saki (rice wine) vinegar and umeboshi (ume) plum vinegar. Add 1/4 tsp. cream of tartar to the bottle for potassium, and these have worked well for sensitive people. You'll just have to try and see. Few people realize that vinegar is a nutrient, and if there's none in the diet, the liver will have to make it.

Keep in mind that vinegar is quite acidic and should be used sparingly, particularly if the urine or saliva pH is in the far acid range (e.g., 5.5 or lower). Note: the ume plum vinegar may actually be alkalizing once it's processed by the body.

People who want to acidify the pH and avoid the viable yeasts in apple cider vinegar can use distilled vinegar. Nutritionists have traditionally shunned distilled vinegar because it lacks the nutrients found in raw vinegars. In this case, however, we're only after the tissue-acidifying effect of the malic acid in the vinegar. Distilled vinegar provides this without the yeast.

Distilled vinegar works well for vinegar douches. Authors of popular candida books who arbitrarily ban vinegar in their candida diets have not looked fully into this subject. There is no yeast in distilled vinegar.

Many of the candida diets restrict sauerkraut, and yet raw sauerkraut shows great promise in its ability to re-seed the G.I. tract with beneficial lactobacillus that can get past the stomach acids. Notice the word "raw." This does not include the canned or pasteurized sauerkrauts. Only recently has a company begun marketing RAW sauerkraut (Vegie Delight) to health food stores. Otherwise you have to make it yourself, which is easy with the right equipment.

The best rejuvalac-type cultures are derived from soaking chopped cabbage overnight and drinking the water. This provides an abundance of living, viable lactobacilli for the health of the G.I. tract. Apple juice and wheat berry cultures have too many viable yeast cells in them. Commercial cultures cost a lot and freeze-dried cultures often die after a few months on the shelf. Yogurt causes excessive mucus and aggravates milk allergies. These facts certainly make drinking a little cabbage water or adding raw sauerkraut look like an intelligent way to boost the lac-bac in the diet.

Candida diet promoters may have gone overboard with their diets, because they have not been able to provide a comprehensive, highly effective program. Many of them are retracting parts of their diets pending further investigation. I've heard that even Dr. Crook, of *The Yeast Connection* fame, has made verbal retractions of his diet plan because it was just a start until further research could be conducted. So be wary of people's attempts to inflict a diet plan on you, particularly if their insights come from popular books. Listen, evaluate, and test it yourself! Read *The Pro Vita! Plan* before embarking upon any dietary adventures.

GENERAL GUIDELINES FROM POPULAR CANDIDA DIETS

Generally, candida diets eliminate sugars. This includes honey, molasses, maple syrup, fructose, and certainly all candies, desserts, fruits, melons, soft drinks, gluten grains (wheat, barley, oats, rye), and chewing gum.

They restrict foods containing yeast, molds, and fungi since these foods cause an immune reaction and reduce a person's resistance to candida. This involves the elimination of breads, beer, wine, dry roasted nuts, and many vinegar foods such as olives, pickles, salad dressings, and soy sauce. Molds are associated with bacon, melons, cheeses, other milk and dairy products (butter is OK, balanced butter is much better), and mushrooms. Check these yourself. Olives may be just fine, but soy sauce not so good. A kinesiologist or electro-acupuncturists can test foods and allergins without expensive, obnoxious skin-reaction tests. Or have a blood work-up.

So what's left? Actually, the candida diet, except for a few difficulties, leaves a very healthy, wholesome, and (with some creativity) delicious meal plan. It is certainly a plan that promotes greater health by all biochemistry standards, if not by the standards of the Standard American Diet —(the sad, S.A.D.) — the one that's been leading us to chronic degenerative diseases with the help of the "four basic food groups" (three of which are represented by powerful lobbies in Washington).

When I asked Stu Wheelwright what a good candida diet was, he gave me a funny look. He said that it's the same low-stress diet he's been teaching for 30 years. Nothing new. A good diet is a good diet regardless of what new disease crops up. He said, "Someday people will catch on. Now the American Heart Association is endorsing a disguised version of this diet and acting like it's something new. Well, I guess it is new in that new research continues to bear out what we've been saying all along." Wheelwright's diet is based on simple food combining, a proper protein matrix, and food values according to their energy ratings.

134

People of all ages who have followed his diet over the last 15 years have flourished and are quick to mention it. The details of this diet are presented in the book, "The Pro-Vita! *Plan*"

There are many surprises to this way of eating — primarily in that it's not too restrictive. Basically, it arranges one or more meals per day to provide balanced protein with a lot of vegetables. Some refer to it as a fish and vegetable meal, but there's more to it than that. As far as I know, it's the only diet that combines insights from biochemistry with insights from quantum chemistry (the science of life energies) to provide a fundamental way of eating for optimal health.

Ultimately it all comes back to diet — the cornerstone of a person's health and one third of the health triad of DIET, EXERCISE, ATTITUDE. Diet plays a crucial role in conquering candida and maintaining a healthy body.

HERBAL SOLUTIONS TO
VIRUS / BACTERIA / FUNGUS

First, let's look at virus — an organism that has eluded medical science for so long. While researchers are still searching for a cure for the common cold, homeopathic medicine offers several formulas that can halt colds in their tracks if they are caught at the right time. One remedy is Anas Barbariae Hepatis et Cordis Extractum HPUS 200 C, which you'll understand if you're versed in Latin. Actually this is a simple remedy that helps the immune system get over the many symptoms of cold virus involvement

. The five major U.S. homeopathic pharmaceutical companies offer natural, effective anti-viral remedies — both as single, classical remedies, and as combination remedies.

Another one, known as "Cold Stop," contains an antivirus factor that can knock colds out at the onset — virtually in one minute. In addition to its antiviral homeopathics, it contains elemental zinc.

Biological medicine already has wonderful remedies for people who are coming down with colds and flus. We really don't need a chemical to accomplish that.

What about the vaccination to prevent colds that medical scientists often talk about? This may not be such a good idea, particularly if colds are a cleansing process that indicates the body is out of balance, instead of a bug that jumps up and grabs people indiscriminately. Medical science may be working on a vaccination that would prevent the natural functioning of the body. We may be fortunate that they've not found a way to conquer the common cold yet.

If a cold is a symptom that our bodies are out of balance, do we want a vaccine that allows us to continue to be out of balance without the symptom of a cold, or would we rathers cleanse, change the cause of imbalance and live a truly healthy life? A vaccine for the cold will only continue the process toward chronic-degeneration, but help people avoid colds in the process.

Leptotoenia

In the herbal kingdom there is an excellent antiviral, antibacterial agent — the wild black carrot, also called leptotoenia or Lomatium disectum. It is quite powerful and supports the immune system in combating colds, flu, herpes (oral and genital), staph infections, and fungal problems. Although it is not a specific for fungus, it does help break the symbiotic relationship between fungus and virus, providing assistance in the fight against fungal infections such as Candidiasis. It has consistently helped people with Epstein-Barr (chronic fatigue) overcome fatigue and live normal lives.

Leptotoenia comes from the wild black carrot, an herb sacred to the Shoshone and Nez Perce Indians. It originally grew in particular regions in Utah, Idaho, Wyoming, and Canada, around the 4500 feet elevation and was a difficult herb to find.

In 1918, the Indians took the oil of leptotoenia to Dr. Krebs (of laetrile fame) in San Francisco during the flu epidemic. It was responsible for saving thousands of lives. This is verified by scientific research.

From the departments of Bacteriology and Chemistry, University of Utah, and the Latter-Day Saints Hospital, Salt Lake City, comes a 6-page report entitled, "Antibiotic Studies on an Extract from Leptotoenia Multifedia," which shows that leptotoenia is comparable to penicillin in its antibacterial activity for a wide variety of infections and many times superior for 12 organisms, including streptococcus, Escherichia coli, pseudomonas, proteus, and particularly effective against acid-fast organisms such astuberculosis. First studies were conducted in 1946 and results were presented at the Second National Symposium on Recent Advances in Antibiotics Research held in Washington, D.C. What's been done about these startling, well-documented findings? They've obviously been ignored for the usual practical reasons — difficulty in supply, inability to standardize, unreliability in harvest, and so forth. Fortunately, herbalists have preserved this knowledge and products such a the Systemic VIVI formula are available through health professionals who feature this miraculous herb.

Leptotoenia has proven itself for colds, herpes, Epstein- Barr, and plays a role in conquering candida by breaking the symbiotic relationship between the virus and the fungus. It helps the body purge itself of the virus, which can strengthen the immune system by relieving it.

Now, let's consider bacteria. Herbology excels in this category, and there are nutritional formulas that can compete head-to-head with many broad-spectrum antibiotics. Only in the most severe case might the chemical drugs be required to simply kill off rampant bacterial invasion in a life or death situation.

Remember that the most natural function of nutrition is PREVENTION, rather than curing serious, chronic diseases after the fact. Since people often wait until the last minute to address health imbalances, nutrition is often called upon to work miracles with chronic and degenerative diseases. A nutritional approach is often very effective in even these difficult cases. With proper attention to nutrition, the body should rarely enter into chronic degenerative states, and acute conditions should be quickly resolved. The need for strong drug medicines should be a rarity.

In most instances, unnatural lifestyles (diet, stress levels, attitudes) create a demand for unnatural chemical drugs to deaden the body's desperate cries to correct itself. So there is a false appearance of health or lack of symptoms called "normality" for a short while until new symptoms appear to remind the body of its unnatural state.

Nutritionists and naturopaths seek to support the body with non-toxic therapies so it can correct imbalances before they become illnesses or diseases. Preventative "medicine" is the keynote which should govern a person's health endeavors rather than "fix it when it breaks".

Goldenseal

While there are many anti-bacterial herbs such as hyssop, yarrow, wild black carrot, raw red potato, echinacea, thyme, tea tree, and hundreds of others, the American (and European-grown) herb goldenseal is unexcelled in its ability to help most people. (Diabetics are an exception as goldenseal is an insulin precursor.)

Unlike antibiotics, which simply kill bacteria, goldenseal stains the harmful bacteria gold, inhibits their reproduction, and clumps them up so the immune system can deal with them.

Goldenseal is innately selective and only works against the harmful bacteria. Unlike antibiotic drugs, it does not harm the beneficial bacteria in the G.I. tract. It works in accord with Nature to enhance the immune system and eliminate bacteria the way the body was designed to work.

This is the fundamental difference between drug therapy and herb therapy. One imposes its will on the body, the other works with the body-systems according to the body's own inherent wisdom.

Goldenseal is best used in conjunction with additional B-complex vitamins. There is an herb formula (GOLD) that combines goldenseal with homeopathic factors, B vitamins, and other herbs, to provide very effective and specific management of bacterial infections — naturally. It's formulas such as these that elevate herbology to new levels of effectiveness, as they are many times more effective than the single herb.

Enough good can't be said about the value of a truly effective, natural antibiotic. And this is the where real grassroots change can occur in the approach to the whole candida problem. If people can overcome bacterial infections without the use of antibiotics, then there is a way to avoid losing what is gained in conquering candida if and when a new bacterial infection occurs. This can mean that there is a way for our children to grow up without ever having to take an antibiotic.

Yarrow

Another herb worth mentioning is yarrow. Recent breakthroughs in the application of this herb show it to be an effective cleanser of subclinical infections when properly combined with other herbs. Oftentimes it is subclinical infections that contribute to the weakened immune system and, thus, these infections become a part the whole candidiasis picture.

Yarrow is a difficult herb to work with because it doesn't combine well with other herbs. It takes special insight to be able to attack subclinical infections by combining yarrow with the proper herbs for deep cleansing and rejuvenation of the immune system. Stu Wheelwright found only a few herbs in the world that could work synergistically with yarrow according to the bio-force principles of its ionization. Research in this area is called ATAK. Most of these compatible herbs come from Brazil and the Amazon valley.

It must be noted that clinical research with the three herbs mentioned here was not done with the individual herb, but with herbal combinations based on the energy pattern of these key herbs. Individually, these herbs do not offer the results that the combinative formulas offer.

Antifungal herbs such as the pau d'arco already discussed exist in nature to balance the fungus kingdom. Since Nature is a balanced and flexible system, somewhere there is a cure for every human ailment in the biological realm. If the research monies being expended on chemical drugs were to be applied to biological, homeopathic, anthroposophical (based on the insights of Rudolph Steiner), eclectic, and herbal research, a new era in genuine health could be manifested. It is unfortunate that the brilliant scientists working to create drugs don't know the first thing about the fascinating and incredibly beautiful "Laws of Nature" that apply to the human biological system. Our understanding of the body could take a quantum leap if only our brilliance were applied to the natural bio-energetic side.

Tea Tree Oil

Australia-produced Tea Tree Oil is a powerful anti-fungal, anti mold spore remedy. It is very effective for topical application to athlete's foot fungus. If alternated with Thymol Iodide (Fanie Thymolize), it can help rid the deep fungus under finger and toenails.

Tea Tree Oil has helped some people get rid of G.I. Tract candida by putting 5 drops in a capsule and taking it with one ounce of Systemic AO (Aloe Vera Concentrate). However, internal use of Tea Tree Oil is contraindicated for people with Epstein Barr (Chronic Fatigue Syndrome) as one of its chemical components can be reactive with the class of virus known as "ghost virus" and cause further complications.

Grapefruit Seed Extract

Extracts from the grapefruit seed are making an impact on the anti mold and fungus market. The extract, which as been available but little known for many years, is now being used in air purifiers, food purifying sprays, and bathroom disinfectants.

The extract is a very potent, natural fungicide, bacteriacide. Wheelwright has incorporated elements of grapefruit seed extracts in his herb formulas and cleansers for many years with excellent results.

More and more we should see this substance incorporated into products to help people de-mold their environment, both external and internal.

A PLAN TO CONQUER CANDIDA

Before jumping into a program, there are some prerequisite considerations. A natural law of the body is that it is biochemically individual. That means that what works for one person may or may not work for another. Individuals will have their own individual responses to the program in terms of die-off reactions, duration, adjunct programs, and the necessary extent of nutritional support.

Furthermore, treatment must often be targeted to each area of infection. So at different times during a program the antifungal therapy may be keyed to the affected areas, such as blood, brain, ears, intestine (large and small), liver, lungs, pancreas, prostate, vagina, and so forth. Constitutional homeopathy offers whole body treatment if the exact remedy can be found. However, success is short-lived (6 months to 2 years) unless the nutritional treatments are also incorporated and the diet supports the work of the remedy.

Constitutional Typing

One additional predetermining factor is a person's constitution. Stu Wheelwright calls this a person's "mannerism," and its classification is based on the size of the blood vessels, tissue integrity, and overall constitution. When he teaches, he refers to these constitutional types as "chickens, lurkeys, and turkeys." The chicken (with small blood vessels) exemplifies the fine-mannered person's constitution and the turkey (with large blood vessels) exemplifies the coarse-mannered person's constitution. The lurkey falls somewhere in-between chickens and a turkeys.

For those readers who are familiar with raising chickens and turkeys, you'll know that the health pattern of chickens is that they are sick and well, sick and well, sick and well, sick and well, and so forth. They respond quickly to treatment (meaning smaller doses are required) and are slow to heal. The health pattern of the turkey is more like well, well, well, well, well, well, sick, dead. They respond slowly to treatment (larger doses are needed) and are quick to heal.

One constitutional type is not necessarily better than another. A chicken may be more sickly, but live longer than a turkey, who may succumb to the first health crisis that comes along.

Of course, people have elements of all three constitutional types in their make-up, but an understanding of the constitutional tendency is critical in choosing your program. As you might expect, chickens require strict diet control, lurkeys just a few changes, and turkeys can usually eat a basically wholesome diet and prosper.

Also, in the case of chicken-types, a therapy should start off very easy with small doses. With turkey-types, a therapy should be more forceful and include larger dosages.

Now to shift from the humorous constitutional type designations to something a bit more respectable, we'll call them Type I, Type II, and Type III, with Type I being fine-mannered chickens, Type II being middle-of-the-road lurkeys, and Type III being coarse-mannered turkeys.

One way to determine constitutional type is by feeling the quality of a person's hair just above the ears. If it is thin, fine, straight hair, it a sign of a Type I. If it is thick, coarse, and (frequently) curly, then it belongs to a Type III. Somewhere in-between is a Type II.

Iridologists, natural health professionals who evaluate health via the markings in the iris of the eye, have an excellent grasp on constitutional types. They can distinguish between them by evaluating the tightness of the fibers in the iris. This is an indication of the collagen strength, which is directly related to constitution. The tighter and straighter the fibers, the stronger the constitution.

Here are a few other pointers for determining constitutional types:

TYPE I

Sensitive (fine-mannered)	TV, movies, candlelight
Reactive	dinners with gourmet foods
Very fine hair	Introspective
Tendency to fashionable	Artistic tendencies
dress	Small blood vessels (can be-
Usually fastidious	come easily clogged)
Enjoys passive activities	Responds quickly, heals slowly
(passive sports/games,	

TYPE II	TYPE III
Average (medium-mannered)	Rugged (coarse-mannered)
Normal hair	Strong, coarse hair
Common skin	Thick skin
Enjoys food of many	Likes bluejeans
varieties (Italian,	Likes active sports
gourmet, western, etc.)	Steak 'n' potatoes people
	Responds slowly, heals quickly

A person's constitutional type has a pronounced bearing on how candida manifests in the body. Type I (fine-mannered) people suffer more but detect it earlier. Their small blood vessels easily become clogged with candida die-off. Type III (coarse-mannered) people can have a little candida in their system without major symptoms.

Three-Step Process

To really conquer candidiasis requires a three-step process:

1. Kill the yeast/fungus and viral parasites and eliminate their toxic wastes from the body. This must be done under the skin, in the G.I Tract, in the bloodstream, in the connective tissue, in the inner-cellular system, in the vagina/prostate, and in any other affected area. This part of the process includes:

A. Stop activities that suppress the immune system, such as using antibiotics, birth control pills, steroids, addictive substances (caffeine, tobacco, sugar). This is a prerequisite for rebuilding the immune system.

B. Alter the diet to eliminate those items that feed yeast thus, inhibiting its further proliferation. Best advice is to follow *The Pro Vita! Diet*.

C. Eliminate symbiotic* parasites (Entamoeba histo-lytica, giardia, protozoa, streptococcus, virus).

This step represents a clean sweep of pathogenic organisms so the immune system gets a rest and can rebuild.

2. Support and rebuild the body's immune system naturally so it can return to its normal function. This step goes hand in hand

with Step 1-A as natural substances may help in the transition from immune-suppressive activities. It means relieving stress and rebuilding of the endocrine glands (thyroid, adrenal, pituitary, thymus) as well as improving the liver function.

3. Re-seed the G.I. tract with a beneficial culture and nourish that culture to continuance through proper diet. Continue to support the immune system. Begin the Liver Triad Program.

It's as simple as that! I know it sounds difficult from the perspective of all the transitional changes required, but all we're doing is returning to the natural state of optimal health, where we ought to be in the first place. We should first understand that we do not really know what natural health is. Most of us only know what artificial health is — a bolstered-up state of feeling OK created by the use of stimulants such as coffee and other drugs that mask the symptoms of what is out of balance. Health is a dynamic state of feeling alive and energetic.

Our bodies were designed to work perfectly. The original blueprint has no flaws. How much of that original blueprint can we manifest in our lives? How much do we want to take the effort to manifest? How much is limited due to genetics congenital defects (birth trauma), accidents, and surgery? These questions form the basis for our health endeavors.

Let's look at Step 1: Kill the fungus. We've discussed the roles of various anticandida/antifungals such as pau d'arco extract, garlic, biotin, zinc, and germanium; short chain fatty acids such as caprylic acid, propionic acid, oleic acid, and extra virgin olive oil; evening primrose oil and flaxseed oil; hydroxyquinoline sulfate acid (from grapefruit rind); Lactobacillus acidophilus and other beneficial cultures such as bifidus, thermophilus, Streptococcus faecium, and bulgaricus; as well as chemistry set items like potassium permanganate, and stabilized oxygen.

The key here is to find the ones that work and do a thorough job. The reversed polarity pau d'arco extract is an excellent place to start. Clinical tests show it helps stop fungus in the bloodstream, thus relieving the immune system. This is verifiable with dark-field microscopy. And it gives some indication of whether or not there will be significant die off reactions, thus letting a person have an idea what the pace should be and whether kidney or colon support is required to help the elimination of toxins.

A homeopathic nosode may help to enhance the body's constitution against infectious yeast/fungus. I recommend professional assistance in using nosode therapy, as I've seen people push the candida in deeper by going through the manufacturer-recommended sequences, which start with low potencies (5X) and then gradually increase to the 200X - 1000X potency. Nosode therapy has only been partially effective. A selection of dietary supplements can supply additional support. Work with a nutritionist/ naturopath to design your first step so it can be effective. This step alone will provide tremendous relief when the candida count is greatly reduced and the toxins removed from the body.

Step 1-A: Eliminate immune-suppressive activities. This is easy for some and difficult for others, depending on the extent that immune suppressive activities are required. A person must not stop an antibiotic in mid-course and must certainly not abandon any prescribed medicine without consulting their doctor. If you are on medication, you must work with your doctor to discontinue it, if it is possible. People hooked on cortisone will have special considerations with which only their doctors can help.

Regularly using medical drugs inhibits the body's ability to respond to nutritional therapies. A lengthy transition period is often required to gradually reduce dependence on drugs and give nutrition the oppurtunity to bring the desired results.

Sugar must be eliminated and other addictive habits reduced and eliminated when possible. It is very difficult to stop all addictions cold turkey because the body is relying on them as an energy source. If you are a heavy user of coffee and cigarettes, you'll probably need the assistance of additional nutritional support as discussed in the book *The Next Step To Greater Energy*.

To continue suppressing the immune system is to go deeper into chronic degenerative disease such as arthritis, diabetes, cancer, AIDS, and osteoporosis. Candida may be your last acute condition, telling you to pull out of your current pattern if you wish to live with any quality.

Step 1-B: Alter the diet to discourage yeast proliferation. All this does is put you back on the diet that promotes health, longevity, vibrancy, and freedom from disease. From that perspective it

146

doesn't seem like such a bad idea, particularly if you have goals for your life or some good reasons to live. Most people find they do not require terribly restrictive diets to be successful in overcoming candida. Basic considerations include: 1) Using fresh vegetables and whole foods, rather than processed and refined products; 2) rotating foods and eating a variety of different foods to avoid allergic reactions; 3) avoiding foods that trigger allergic reactions and sensitivities; and 4) avoiding overeating, which taxes the whole body.

Step 1-C: Eliminate symbiotic* parasites (Entamoeba histolytica, giardia, protozoa, streptococcus, virus). It seems that when trouble comes, it comes in legions. If one microorganism overrides the immune system, others get in as well. The Epstein-Barr virus (a relative of mononucleosis) is particularly symbiotic* with candida. Some people go on antifungus programs, but do not respond with the success that others have. In such cases, other microorganisms should be suspected.

We've already mentioned the candida-virus connection. And there are others, such as giardia, a protozoan that is increasingly bothersome. Giardia is competitive with candida. It is possible that when candida is reduced in the body, giardia can proliferate, and vice versa. If both are suspected, both must be treated.

Also, candida seems to encourage streptococcus proliferation. The streptococcus probably finds a food source in the by-products of the cell-invasive fungal action.

Recent research from England links streptococcus with osteoarthritis. Evidently one way the body defends itself against streptococcus is by encasing it in calcium. This calcium can build up in joints, tissues, and weakened areas of the body.

Amoebas are also implicated in arthritis by the same process. Several medical doctors have built their reputations on prescribing Flagyl (an anti-amoeba drug) for arthritis. [Note: Flagyl is a very toxic drug with many side effects.]

There are natural, effective herbal and homeopathic solutions to the microorganism problem, and, once they are eliminated, the body's immune system can be strengthened nutritionally, so it can return to its natural function.

Step 2: Support the immune system. This is important since the diet aims to avoid allergins such as food containing yeast, mold, and fungi as well as foods that cause sensitivities. Immune system supports also include supplements, because by the time people have candidiasis their immune systems need specific support to turn around and become stronger. Natural support of the immune system means focusing on herbs, minerals, and herbal formulas that help control bacteria, yeast, and subclinical infections. We discussed goldenseal, echinacea, and yarrow-based research that investigates ways to attack subclinical infections, and also talked about homeopathic nosodes* as ways of building up the immune system by flushing out the disease. Antioxidant minerals (germanium, zinc, selenium) provide direct immune support.

Many researchers are studying the role of the thymus gland in the body's immune response. Nutritional support of the thymus may be an important factor in overcoming a variety of conditions such as herpes, allergies, asthma, and so forth. Nutritional support of the thymus is important in any candida program.

Step 3: Re-seed the G.I. tract. Working with the various beneficial bacteria cultures is about the best thing a person can do at this time. A diet that focuses on vegetables and ample dietary fiber helps reestablish a more proper intestinal flora. Also, there are herb formulas that help the small intestine heal where the fungus attacked the mucosa. It is essential to repair the G.I. tract to help stop the food allergies. Once repaired, the undigested proteins and foods will not be absorbed too soon and cause so many allergic reactions. This is a big step in helping to relieve the immune system as well.

Once a person is stable in their return to health, raw sauerkraut offers an effective way to support the intestinal culture dietarily without resorting to dairy products such as yogurt.

Each of these steps is interwoven with the others and the success of the whole program depends, to some extent on each of the other parts. This is the most comprehensive program available today, as it works to solve the problem of candida on every front: nutritionally, biochemically, attitudinally, and bio-energetically.

The Immune System Support Program (Example)

This plan for conquering candida is based on clinical research that has resulted in the most profound benefits of any program to date. Research and case history documentation continues, but these guidelines are provided to doctors and health professionals now, so they may implement this truly effective, nutritional program without delay.

It is not possible to design one program for all people. Fine-mannered people will proceed with caution lest they encounter "die-off" reactions, but coarse-mannered people will plow right through this program. Some will require eliminative support (kidneys, bowels). Others will not. Some will require close compliance with dietary recommendations, others not so much. But if people follow the **concept** of this program, they too will earn a greater degree of total health based on the more optimal functioning of the body's systems.

This is an herbal-formula program that deals directly with candidiasis. This program represents Step 1 and part of Step 2. In addition to this basic program, consideration must be given to focusing the program on target areas, i.e., prostate, vagina, liver, lungs, brain, and so forth. Special attention should be paid to the skin (subcutaneous candidiasis) by using Sweet Birch cleanser instead of soap as already mentioned. The formula codes are included for doctors already familiar with their applications.

Note: This is a general program. Your doctor or nutritionist can tailor this program to your specific constitutional type, your gender, and to your particular case of candidiasis. Additional supports to assist detoxification, overall nutrition, diet parameters, endocrine gland function, liver system function, and the elimination of symbiotic organisms will be programmed by your health professional.

Since specific formulas are referred to, and people have vested interests in the sale of products, this disclaimer is provided:

This information is restricted to professional use. No statement contained herein shall be construed as a claim or representation that any product constitutes either specific cure, palliative, or ameliorative for any condition of ill health. This information is not intended as labeling for any product, nor shall it be employed by anyone as labeling. Certain persons considered experts may disagree with one or more of the conclusions and opinions reported herein, but they are nevertheless deemed to be of current nutritional interest and to be based upon reliable and sound authority in the author's best judgment.

1 Bifivia, every day, throughout program.

Days 1 to 3:   1 drop Tai-Ra-Chi in 4 ounces water
1 #4 (Corrector) — away from food and other supplements
Vaginal douche: Add 1 tbsp. XL and 3 drops Tai-Ra-Chi to a pint of pure water. Then add 1 capsule #4 (Corrector) and stir. Douche one time a day for 10 days. Retain as able. Begin the Pro-Vita! Diet.

Days 4 to 6:   2 drops Tai-Ra-Chi — two times a day
1 #4 (Corrector) — two times a day
Adjunctive therapies: begin caprylic acid, garlic, cultures, etc. if desired.

Days 7 to 12:   3 drops Tai-Ra-Chi — two times a day
2 #4 (Corrector) — two times a day
Adjunctive therapies: begin nosodes.

Days 13 to 24: 6 drops Tai-Ra-Chi — three times a day
2 #4 (Corrector) plus 1 VIVI (Anti Viro)— two times a day,
1 ATAK
Adjunctive therapies: begin alternating acidophilus, bifidus cultures. Add raw sauerkraut to diet if not already begun.

Days 25 to 40: 6 drops Tai-Ra-Chi — three times a day
2 #4 (Corrector) — two times a day
1 ATAK plus 1 VIVI — four times a day
Adjunctive therapy: begin germanium supplementation or injections.

Days 41 to 75:   6 drops Tai-Ra-Chi — three times a day
                  2 #4 (Corrector) plus
                  1 VIVI (Anti Viro)—4 times a day
                  1 ATAK —four times a day
                  2 P (Pancreas) —early in the day
                  1 Gt (Thymus) —in mid-afternoon

Day 76 on: For 10 days: 1 #4 (Corrector) per day
                  1 Gt two times a day,

Then for the next 10 days: 1 ATAK per day and 1 Gt two times a
                  day,

Then for the 3rd 10 days: 1 VIVI per day

Repeat the rotation of Day 76 on. Begin Liver Triad program.

Each person's pattern or relationship with candida is unique. It is important to choose just the right supplements. This is where a nutritional counselor becomes quite valuable. One of the greatest shortcomings of the medical model is that it treats all people the same — the same drug causing the same chemical reaction, as if all people can be reduced to a single test tube. If you choose natural means of conquering candida, your program will be tailored to your specific needs. There are choices to be made each step of the way regarding which formulas are best for you.

People need to understand that technology isn't the answer to health problems. It's a valuable tool, but Nature is the healer, and the body is built from an organic, living blueprint. Chemical drugs cover symptoms, suppress disease, and hurt other areas of the body. Herbs, like the body, are built from an organic, living blueprint and can heal without harming other areas of the body.

If, however, you use this material and design your own program to include elements of each of the three steps and you choose good quality formulas that really work, you'll find tremendous success in overcoming the debilitating effects of candidiasis.

The time it takes is determined by how fast people can go, by the quality of nutritional supports, how much die-off is experienced, and how committed a person is to working a comprehensive program. Anyone can get relief with either nutrition or drugs. But to conquer candida takes a concerted effort and discipline. Nutrition is the only field right now providing people with a pathway to regain health and keep it. But that only makes sense. Nutrition (including light, air, foods, exercise, and connection with the Vital Force) is the only natural pathway we have for physical health.

Included are program sheets for your health professional to use to outline your specific nutritional program.

Best wishes in all your health endeavors!

STRESS CONTROL NUTRITIONAL PROGRAM

NAME _____ DATE _____ PROGRAM #_____ FOR _____ DAYS

These are foods for dietary use only and are in accordance with the Proxmire-Delany Amendment, 1975. Results are nutritional only. This is not a prescription

UPON ARISING	30 MIN. AFTER ARISING	WITH BREAKFAST (PRO-VITA! 5 + 5)	MID MORNING (Away from food)
12 oz. pure water			12 oz. pure water

20 MIN. BEFORE LUNCH	WITH LUNCH	MID AFTERNOON (Away from food)	20 MIN. BEFORE SUPPER
		12 oz. pure water	

WITH SUPPER	30 MIN. BEFORE BED	BEFORE BED	EDUCATION/READ:
	8 oz. pure water		_____ Conquer Candida
			_____ Energy & Addictions
			_____ Herbs
			_____ Homeopathy
			_____ Liver Triad
			_____ Pro Vita! Diet

A. Drops _____ _____ dropper _____x/day B. Drops _____ _____ dropper _____x/day
C. _____
D. _____

Schedule: _____ Clinic Blood Screen, _____ Clinic Urinalysis _____ Blood Lab Tests _____
_____ Amino Acid Profile, _____ Hair/Tissue Analysis, _____ Stool Test, _____ Lung Test, _____ Allergins
Schedule Follow Up Test _____ in _____ days

Notes:
1. Increase daily water intake by 42 oz. (4 additional glasses), follow diet plan.
2. Use of the following items will reduce the effectiveness of this program and should be avoided: head (iceberg) lettuce [use leaf lettuce instead], margarine [use real butter sparingly instead], soft drinks (including Nutrasweet, diet, and caffeine-free soft drinks), tobacco, alcoholic drinks, foods cooked in aluminum cookware, coffee, pekoe tea, recreational drugs (marijuana), refined sugar products and fried foods. Substitute with wholesome, living foods. Best wishes in your health endeavors!
3. Follow this program for 6 days, leave off the 7th day. Begin again for 6 days. Rest on the 7th day, etc.

153

STRESS CONTROL NUTRITIONAL PROGRAM

Name _____ Date _____

These are foods for dietary use only and are in accordance with the Proxmire-Delany Amendment, 1975. Results are nutritional only. This is not a prescription.

PROGRAM #1 FOR DAYS 1 - 30	PROGRAM #2 FOR DAYS 31 - 60	PROGRAM #3 FOR DAYS 61 - 90
Upon Arising _____	Upon Arising _____	Upon Arising _____
20 Min. Later _____	20 Min. Later _____	20 Min. Later _____
10 Min. Before Breakfast _____	10 Min. Before Breakfast _____	10 Min. Before Breakfast _____
With Breakfast _____	With Breakfast _____	With Breakfast _____
Mid Morning (2 hr. after food)	Mid Morning (2 hr. after food)	Mid Morning (2 hr. after food)
20 Min. Later _____	20 Min. Later _____	20 Min. Later _____
10 Min Before Lunch _____	10 Min. Before Lunch _____	10 Min. Before Lunch _____
With Lunch _____	With Lunch _____	With Lunch _____
Mid Afternoon - 2 hr. from food	Mid Afternoon - 2 hr. from food	Mid Afternoon - 2 hr. from food
30 Min. Later _____	30 Min. Later _____	30 Min. Later _____
10 Min. Before Supper _____	10 Min. Before Supper _____	10 Min. Before Supper _____
With Supper _____	With Supper _____	With Supper _____
30 Min. Before Bed _____	30 Min. Before Bed _____	30 Min. Before Bed _____
Before Bed _____	Before Bed _____	Before Bed _____

Note: Increase water intake by 36 oz./day. Use of the following items will reduce the effectiveness of the program and should be avoided: head (iceberg) lettuce (use leaf lettuce), margarine (use real butter sparingly), soft drinks (including nutrasweet), alcoholic drinks, foods cooked in aluminum cookware, coffee, pekoe tea.

154

TREATING YOUR FOODS TO RID THEM OF POISONOUS SPRAYS, BACTERIA, FUNGI, AND HEAVY METALS

As you know, most of our produce is laced with insecticides and chemical fertilizers, gassed to induce ripening, and treated to preserve shelf-life. Furthermore, industrial wastes are turning up in agricultural water and end up in the plants. In addition to that, produce often has molds, fungi, and parasites, or parasite eggs on it.

There is a simple procedure to protect yourself and your family from this, and it should be used before any produce goes into your refrigerator. It's called the CHLOROX SOAK or the HYDROGEN PEROXIDE (H2O2) SOAK. And basically it means to soak all your fruits, vegetables, eggs, and meats in a Chlorox or H2O2 solution for a few minutes. Frozen meats may be soaked later, except ground meat, which does not have a suitable texture.

Note: an extract from fermented grapefruit seed such as Systemic's XL formula can also be used. The grapefruit seed extract contains a powerful antifungal, anti-candida, anti-mold, anti-bacterial agent. But nothing yet to be found works as well and costs as little as simple Chlorox, plain, unscented.

There are many advantages to this treatment: Fruits and vegetables will keep much longer before molding or wilting, flavors are improved, color is improved, nutritional value will not be compromised, and you will not end up eating chlorine or peroxide.

Note: Regarding eggs — this is a soak, not a scrubbing. The viscid coating on eggs (provided by the hen) protects the eggs and should not be scrubbed off. Just soak the eggs and let them dry.

Here's the procedure:

Use only Chlorox — the regular Chlorox bleach — not any other brand. Only Chlorox is made in stainless steel containers and bottled without the opportunity for oxidation with the plastic bottle.

Upon opening the bottle, it is best to transfer the Chlorox to a glass container so there is no oxidative reaction with the plastic container after it is opened.

155

Use one teaspoon of Chlorox to one gallon of cool tap water in your sink. Into this bath place your fruits, vegetables, eggs, and meat. Note: Using more Chlorox is not better.

This procedure makes something similar to a homeopathic potentization of the Chlorox. The action of the Chlorox is said to be magnetic, which means that its strong negative charge will pull the toxin's positively charged molecules out of the produce. Too much Chlorox can cause oxidative damage to tender vegetables (sprouts, etc.), so measure accurately. For people who are chlorine-sensitive (environmentally sensitive), a solution of hydrogen peroxide (H_2O_2) will accomplish much of what the Chlorox can do.

People who prefer the hydrogen peroxide soak usually use the 35% food grade H_2O_2 and dilute it to 1% with the water in the sink.

The general time of soaking is 10 minutes. Leafy vegetables and thin-skinned fruits will require 10 minutes. Roots, eggs, and meats will require 15 minutes. Do not leave items in longer than 15 or 20 minutes.

Some people separate their produce into 4 categories and soak them separately. The categories are: 1) Vegetables, sprouts, apples, peaches, bananas, and citrus; 2) roots and potatoes; 3) eggs; and 4) meats. Freshen the soak solution each time.

Soaking times increase accordingly: Category one is 10 minutes. Category four is 15 minutes.

Note: People often forget to soak their eggs. Eggs rate very high as an allergy-causing food, due to the pesticide sprays used around the pens. Eggshell is actually very porous and eggs can absorb many toxic sprays from their environment. Salmonella bacteria is also usually present in the egg. By soaking eggs in the Chlorox bath for 15 minutes, you will find they have a better flavor and, when cooked properly at 180 to 200 degrees F, they lose their tendency to create allergies.

After the produce soaks in the Chlorox or H_2O_2 solution, then soak it in the tap water for 10 minutes to remove any Chlorox. Then rinse under the tap and lay out on a terry cloth towel to dry. When dry, put in food storage containers, and then into the refrigerator.

Many people cut the ends off celery and lettuce before soaking so each stalk and leaf can soak and be cleaned prior to putting them into the refrigerator. This furnishes a ready supply of salad and snack materials.

Meats need to soak the longest time as they are carriers of many toxic materials, including antibiotic shots, steroids, drugs, sprays, and ingested toxins. Fish can have a high mercury content and simply soaking helps remove some of these toxic substances. The magnetic action caused by the Chlorox pulls some of the heavy metals out of produce.

Chlorox soaking of all produce should become a standard procedure for your home. There are many seemingly incurable conditions affecting people today, all caused by the massive accumulation of environmental poisons.

This is a simple safeguard to avoid many of the sprays, metallics, and insecticides, as well as bacteria and fungus.

AFTERWORD

Since this information is based on clinical testing, we often get letters asking, "What are good brands of acidophilus?" or "Should germanium be sublingual?" or "Where do I get non-soap shampoo?" and so forth. In our testing we found distinct differences in the healing abilities of supplements.

For instance, we tested 32 brands of cultures (acidophilus, bifidus, etc.) and have distinct preferences for certain ones that have proven themselves clinically effective.

The publisher has agreed to provide a list of the best formulas (as they are known today — the list changes occasionally as research continues). The list features products from many vendors and all entries are unsolicited. All products listed are basically "over the counter". Professional products — those requiring the guidance or administration of a health professional - are not listed. To receive the list, send a stamped, self-addressed envelope to the publisher.

Apple-A-Day...Press

1500 Village West #77
Austin, Texas 78733-1977
apple-a-day@austin.rr.com
www.apple-a-daypress.com

GLOSSARY

AMINO ACID: Any of a class of organic compounds containing the amino group NH2. Amino acids are the primary structures of proteins. Currently there are eight known essential amino acids that are not manufactured by the body and must be obtained through diet. A ninth may soon be recognized. The other 14 or so nonessential amino acids can be manufactured by the body (a function of the liver) from the available essential amino acids in the body.

ANTIBODY: A protein molecule with a specific amino acid sequence produced in response to the presence of foreign (antigenic) substances in the body. Antibodies bind to their specific antigen like a key fits a lock and are only effective when the key fits. Antibodies are responsible for the body's immune response to thousands of potentiallydamaging diseases.

BIOLOGICAL MEDICINES: Nutrients, herbs, homeopathics that support the whole, living body system. [As opposed to allopathic medicines, which are usually chemically, synthetically derived and counteract symptoms.]

CANDIDA ALBICANS: A yeast-like microorganism normally present in human beings in a workable relationship to other bacteria cultures. When the environment is disturbed, it has the ability to infect healthy tissue via its fungal form.

CANDIDIASIS: Pathogenic yeast/fungus overgrowth. The disease caused by cell-invasive Candida albicans.

DYSBIOSIS: A condition where there is a greater number of pathogenic microorganisms inhabiting the gastrointestinal tract than there are beneficial ones.

HOMEOPATHY: A system of medicine founded by Samuel Hahnemann in the late 18th Century that utilizes minute dosages of substances that cause similar symptoms in a healthy individual. One basic premise is "Like cures like." Homeopathic medicines are nonpoisonous, safe, inexpensive, extremely effective, and actively suppressed in the United States by the pharmaceutical companies and the American Medical Association. They are used by the medical profession throughout the rest of the world with great success.

HOMEOPATHIC NOSODE: A potentization (scientifically-prepared dilution) of the disease itself, used to assist the body in bringing it up and throwing it off. Like cures like. A tiny portion of a disease such as syphilis can be potentized, even beyond the point where there is any physical remnant of the disease left, and cause the body to heal itself of that disease when injected or taken orally (or when it comes into contact with any mucous membrane). Nosodes, because they are specific remedies for the disease itself made from the disease itself, can be used kinesiologically to better determine the exact cause of a person's discomfort.

IN VITRO: Studies conducted outside the body in an artificial environment such as a test tube.

IN VIVO: Studies conducted in living bodies (plant, animal, human).

NATUROPATHY: The caring for and healing of the body according to natural laws and natural methods. Naturopathic physicians often employ homeopathy, herbology, acupuncture, diet, clinical nutrition, massage, and reflexology as tools to restore and maintain health. The principles of Naturopathic healing are 1) Rely on the healing power of nature, 2) Treat the whole person (not just the symptoms), 3) Do no harm, 4) Identify and treat the cause, 5) Prevention is the best cure, 6) The doctor is a teacher.

PANDEMIC: A widespread epidemic disease distributed throughout at least a continent and may even be global.

PATHOGEN: A microorganism or substance that is capable of producing disease.

PROTOMORPHAGENS: Extracts of animal organ tissues containing the genetic structure of that organ. Used with herbs, they can provide a matrix for more specific directing of the herbal healing influences.

SYMBIOTIC: The intimate living together of two dissimilar organisms in a mutually beneficial relationship.

SYSTEMIC: Affecting the body as a whole.

ABOUT THE AUTHOR

Jack Tips, ND, PhD, brings the message of dynamic, vital health to thousands of people through lectures, seminars, articles, radio, books, television and clinical practice. *"Health is a dynamic state wherein the body, the emotions, and the mind are bio-energetically in accord with the flow of Life Force, expressing adaptability, vitality, and joy."*

Beginning in 1971, his background includes personal studies with many of the world's renowned health leaders: Dr. Bernard Jensen (iridology, naturopathy), Dr. Wilhelm Langreder (German nosode homeopathy), Dr. A.S. Wheelwright (systemic herbology, bioenergetic nutrition, sclerology), Stanley Burroughs (cleansing, color therapy), Dr. Francisco Eizayaga (clinical homeopathy), Dr. Paul Eck (tissue mineral ratios), Dr. Alan Beardall (kinesiology), Dr. Herbert Shelton (fasting, hygiene), and Dr. Robin Murphy (classical homeopathy). He also studied at the Occidental Institute Research Foundation (electro-acupuncture, vega-test, Mora therapy) in Vancouver, BC.

In 1980, Dr. Tips began consulting in the applications of systemic herbology, homeopathy and clinical nutrition. He earned a PhD in Nutrition Science from Clayton University (The Dr. Roger Williams School of Nutrition Science), and an ND (Doctorate of Naturopathy — a 2 year curriculum) from Clayton University in Clayton, Missouri. His dissertation, published as *Conquer Candida and Restore Your Immune System* has received international recognition as a definitive work on the philosophy of natural cure and the challenges of the immune system. He has also authored *The Next Step to Greater Energy, Your Liver...Your Lifeline,* and *The Art and Science of Sclerology, Blood Chemistry & Clinical Nutrition,* as well as numerous articles on women's health. He holds a Fellowship in the American Council of Applied Clinical Nutrition (FACACN), and is certified as a Nutritional Consultant (CNC) by the American Council of Nutrition Consultants. He serves on the board of directors of the Texas chapter of the International and American Association of Clinical Nutritionists. He is registered as a practicing homeopath with the National Center for Homeopathy, Washington, DC, and is a member of the International Foundation for Homeopathy; the Homeopathic Academy of Naturopathic Physicians, and graduate of and active participant with the Hahnemann Academy of North America (CHom).

In 1993, he became a minister for Life Resources, an integrated auxiliary of Freedom Church of Revelation, and established his ministry through Apple-A-Day. His ministry is dedicated to the healing of the whole person with natural methods.

Currently, he is president of the International Sclerology Foundation, teacher with the Westlake Homeopathic Society, and director of the Apple-A-Day Clinic, Austin, Texas, where he consults with individuals, both in person and by phone. He resides in Austin with his wife, children, and step children. Dr. Tips is dedicated to providing people the knowledge and tools to live genuinely healthy lives.

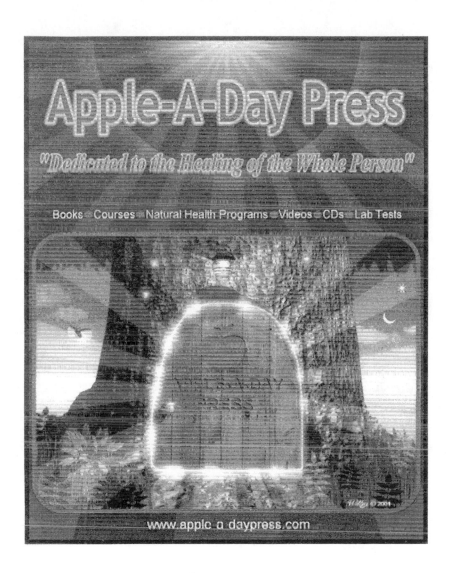

Apple-A-Day Press
1500 Village West Drive, Suite 77
Austin, TX 78733

Phone: 512-328-3996
Toll Free: 877-442-7753
Fax: 512-263-7787
E-mail: apple-a-day@austin.rr.com

Welcome to Apple-A-Day Press: Your natural health resource!

Here you'll find some of the most amazing and informative books, courses, and healing programs available in the world today!

Since 1984, Apple-A-Day Press has published insightful books and natural health courses that have helped thousands (even millions) of people with their health. With a primary focus on the research and writings of Dr. Jack Tips, nothing here is like what you've encountered before. At Apple-A-Day, you'll view health and healing from a totally new perspective—one that is deeper (the ancient wisdom of the historical research), wider ('horse sense' makes a lot of sense with health!), more well-rounded (the insights of experience), and watch out—you may catch a dose of dry Texas humor! These books are jam-packed with valuable information that truly brings the gift of health.

You'll find much more information on our web site, www.apple-a-daypress.com including downloads of chapters of our books, other free articles, lab tests, nutritional programs, and health building tools.

It is indeed an honor and a pleasure to share these tools, insights and knowledge with you. It is our foremost desire that this site contribute to your good health, good insight, and good life...Best Wishes in your health endeavors!

Apple-A-Day Press

Toll free order line: 1-877-442-7753
(orders only, 24-hours secure)

Or on-line: www.apple-a-daypress.com

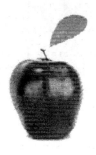

Natural Healing at Your Fingertips

For more information on your "do it yourself" health improvement system, log on to www.apple-a-daypress.com.

Join the Apple-A-Day Press confidential mailing list and be the first to know about new books, discounts, special offers and seminars. Join on line at www.apple-a-daypress.com or phone or fax a note.

APPLE-A-DAY PRESS

1500 Village West Drive, Suite 77, Austin, Texas, 78733
Phone: 512.328.3996 Fax: 512.263.7787
Website: www.apple-a-daypress.com
Email: apple-a-day@austin.rr.com

Passion Play

by Dr. Jack Tips

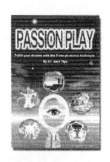

If ever a book could change your life—increase your wealth, improve your relationships, and open your heart—this is it. Absolutely profound and insightful. Believe this—the Mirror Technique is a true shortcut to success in any endeavor. It starts where other self-help books leave off—beyond affirmations, beyond visualization, beyond anything you've ever tried!

Passion Play is the art of combining Sensualization with the Native American Mirror Technique to harness your hidden power of manifestation. Use this technique to awaken your heart, encourage your actions, enliven your dreams, clarify your mission, achieve your goals and discover your true destiny. Passion Play is a new, powerful breakthrough in self-realization and human potential. Wealth, love, romance, success, charity, health, freedom, contentment, joy, excitement and spiritual adventures await you—within these pages, within your life. Never before has the step-by-step process to recreate yourself, create your future life, and follow your heart's desire become so clear, simple, and effective. Now you can discover your passion and begin your play. Passion Play will improve your life—Forever.

333 pages   ISBN 0-929167-20-1 $21.95

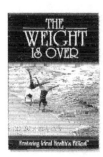

The Weight Is Over

by Dr. Jack Tips

A powerful, health-building book. The last weight-loss book you'll ever need! Much more than how to lose weight, this book teaches how to gain true health! Anyone can benefit from this myth-busting breakthrough!

Get trim now! It's not your fault your weight is up and your energy is down. You've avoided fat, you've increased grains, you've eaten less—just like they told you. But you know what? They told you wrong! Now, for the first time, find out why people have excessive weight and how you can eradicate it. Learn about the perfect custom-designed eating plan for you as an individual! Take The FitTest—a simple, in-home lab test that reveals how to get trim now. The Weight Is Over is a groundbreaking new program that takes you step by step into a mastery of nutrition—both eating to lose fat and building optimal health simultaneously. Much more than a crash program, this book helps you build a healthy lifestyle that will benefit you for the rest of your life. Learn about:

- So called "bad" foods that are really good for you!
- Super foods that unleash your body's ability to burn fat while you sleep!
- Herbs and nutrients that help you burn fat for energy!
- 'Syndrome X' and how it silently kills people.
- The 12 Optimal Food Factors never before published insights on everything your diet must provide you to prevent disease and be healthy!

The Weight Is Over is more than guidelines and tips, it is a strategic action plan, based on over 30-years of research and clinical experience. You'll be taken through the maze of nutrition confusion into a very simple, crystal clear program that brings you success you can keep. It's easy, it's fun, it's effective!

Hardback - 300 pages (limited edition)   ISBN 0-929167-19-8 $27.95
Paperback (available October, 2001)   ISBN 0-929167-21-X $21.95

The Pro-Vita! Plan
for Optimal Nutrition
by Dr. Jack Tips

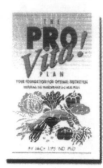

A nutrition classic and one of the most important natural health books of the 20th Century! Absolutely a must read for every natural health practitioner and anyone wanting to end the confusion about dietary health.

Here is a simple and comprehensive way to build your health, prevent disease, and increase longevity based on both biochemistry and bio-energy! An extraordinary overview of how to minimize dietary stress and maximize utilization of the highest quality food factors: protein, fat, carbohydrates, minerals, vitamins, enzymes, fiber, and nascent water, and bio-energy.

A safe, non-radical nutritional foundation based on the 'ancient wisdom' and 'common sense' that can change your life and bring the best of health.

Daily nutrition plans and delicious recipes are included. Learn how to design the optimal nutrition meal and turn your eating experience into a healing experience! You will gain a greater understanding of nutrition and its role in health. A simple approach to more energy, weight loss, improved immunity, and better health!

376 pages, index   ISBN 0-929167-05-8   **$21.95**

To order, call toll free: 1-877-442-7753
Or go on-line: www.apple-a-daypress.com

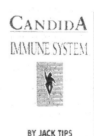

Conquer Candida—Restore
Your Immune System
by Dr. Jack Tips

Not just another candida book but a natural health milestone. This book goes where others have never dared— a deeper understanding of health and its restoration.

Hailed by readers and natural health practitioners alike as the finest and most easy to understand book about the "canary in the mine shaft" regarding your health. Not just another candida book, here is an in-depth look at the silent, health-undermining pandemic that contributes to allergies, chronic fatigue, PMS, chronic infections, headaches, bloating, memory loss, and immune deficiencies. More importantly, this book explains what to do about these conditions by indicating true causes and offering unique insights based on hundreds of clinical case histories. "Many people blame all their health ailments on candida (yeast fungus), but this is not really the problem! Many people overlook the fact that candida is not only a symptom of impaired immunity, it also predisposes people to further poor health and low energy. You cannot quickly win the battle against candida by dietary adjustment, but you can with proper natural health therapy." Find out if candida is a factor in your health picture and what to do about it with the Apple-A-Day comprehensive program. This information goes beyond current treatments and offers an understanding of how to truly conquer candida and restore your most optimal health.

163 pages   ISBN 0-929167-00-7   **$15.95**

Breast Health – A Women's Health Discourse
by Dr. Jack Tips

Are you simply waiting and hoping your next mammogram won't steal your life with the dreaded news? Find out what you can do now to not only protect your health but to have overall female hormone balance. Find out why men need to read this material.

From the natural health perspective, there are clear reasons that breast cancer occurs and thus there are clear steps to take to prevent it! In this discourse, you will learn the reasons that the breast tissue is susceptible to disease and learn simple steps to avoid them. Beyond disease concerns, the breasts play an important role in overall female hormonal balance. Breast health is an important part of overcoming PMS, menstrual cramping, endometriosis, and menopausal symptoms. This discourse discusses the role of breast tissue in female endocrine balance and demonstrates how to maintain healthy breast tissue. Features the breast-test and breast massage technique to help prevent breast disease and maintain tissue integrity.

56 pages, illustrations **$8.95**

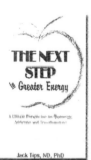

The Next Step to Greater Energy: A Unique Perspective on Bioenergy, Addictions and Transformation
by Dr. Jack Tips

Are your "little addictions" a clear symptom of a metabolic imbalance? Breaking addictive behaviors is more effective with this information.

Explore the energy systems of the body with emphasis on both the glandular (thyroid and adrenals) and bio-electric energy systems. This book presents a new look at the connection between bio-energy and addictions. Discover energy impostors including substances, activities, and habits. Identify addictions and habits as symptoms of bio-energetic and biochemical imbalances. Discover the true cause of cravings and addictive patterns, and how to correct the underlying imbalances. How to stop smoking is thoroughly discussed. The focus of this practical information is how to obtain freedom and fuller spiritual expression.

210 pages, index   ISBN 0-929167-04-X **$16.95**

WOMEN'S HEALTH DISCOURSES BY DR. JACK TIPS

Formerly available for sale in this catalog, the discourses on Menopause, PMS, and Osteoporosis among many others are now available for free on the website www.jacktips.com. Enjoy the gift of health-empowering information from Dr. Tips!

Your Liver–Your Lifeline!   by Dr. Jack Tips

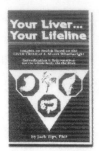

The liver—the most important organ in your body and a key part of your immune system. Fascinating insights on how to detoxify your entire body by building your inherent liver function. This information changes lives!

Featured at Anthony Robbins' Life Mastery University, here is the key to detoxification and restoration of proper liver function. This is a fascinating look at the liver—your most important organ—its bioforces and the Chinese healing system involving the triad of the liver-stomach-colon. Explains in easy steps how to detoxify your liver, gall bladder and entire body the natural way. Contains provocative insights into how herbs really work to help your body heal. Reveals natural liver treatments and cures. Shows you how to build the very foundation upon which your health rests! Doc Wheelwright discovered seven herbs that he called "miraculous" that support the complex liver systems and created a remarkable breakthrough in liver support. A must read for people with concerns regarding Hepatitis C and anyone wanting to live life in the best of health.

150 pages, illustrations, photos, index   ISBN 0-929167-06-6 $14.95

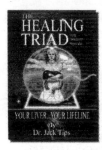

The Healing Triad (CD's)   with Dr. Jack Tips

A candid discussion on the ancient Chinese foundation of healing and the 21st Century applications brought forth by Doc Wheelwright.

Master vibrant health in a polluted world! Learn about the ancient healing triad, the truth about parasites, and a simple technique for detecting liver problems. Find out about the liver's role in allergies, PMS, candida, fatigue, and skin problems. In this lively discussion, you'll discover how to improve digestion, detoxification and elimination.

2 CD set in binder   ISBN 0-929167-13-9 $19.95

To order, call toll free: 1-877-442-7753
Or go on-line: www.apple-a-daypress.com

Cooking with Brooke
Recipes   by Melane Lohmann

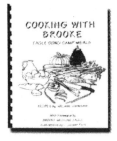

Wonderful, healthful Pro-Vita! Recipes from a wonderful cook.

Delicious Pro-Vita! Recipes served by Brooke Medicine Eagle at the Eagle Song Camp (Blacktail Ranch, Montana). A great companion of simple, tasty recipes based on the *Pro-Vita! Plan For Optimal Nutrition*.

57 pages, spiral bound, illustrated $11.00

A Guidebook to Clinical Nutrition for the Health Professional

by Dr. Timothy Kuss

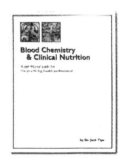

What to do and how to do it. Valuable information on how to help people heal.

A fascinating guide and desk reference through Dr. Wheelwright's work with herbs by one of his leading protégés. Includes a 400-entry Clinician's Manual of herbal protocols, and demonstrates Dr. Wheelwright's bioenergetic research. Full of valuable information on the natural cure of the most common health concerns. Includes more than the Wheelwright herbal system and embraces the full spectrum of natural healing.

For additional health professional offerings, please visit www.jacktips.com

Revised in 2001, 275 pages $21.95

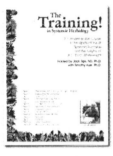

Systemic Nutrition/Herbology Training Program (The Training!)

by Dr. Jack Tips with Dr. Tim Kuss

Master the Doc Wheelwright healing formulas and learn his programming secrets with this cassette course that becomes your desk reference book for one of the most advanced healing systems in the world.

For the health professional, this training program features 14 cassette tapes, a discourse on advanced applications of Doc Wheelwright's herbal system, and a 200-page desk reference for thorough training in the applications of Wheelwright's research and Systemic Herbal Formulas. Reveals Wheelwright's secrets about how and why he created his famous herbal healing combinations. You will quickly become proficient in comprehensive program design using Wheelwright's complete healing system. This program will make you a master of systemic herbology. (*The Training* is a prerequisite for the Health Professionals' 2nd Opinion Program.)

14 cassettes in binder, discourse (protocols), 200-page manual $159.00

Blood Chemistry & Clinical Nutrition

by Dr. Jack Tips

Deep nutritional insights from the ordinary Auto-Chem, SMAC-26/CBC blood test.

For the clinical nutritionist, this manual and desk reference examines each blood test value from the SMAC-26/CBC lab test for its nutritional health implications and provides Systemic Formulas protocols for correcting imbalances. Includes optimal values, pathologies, clinical notes, cross-references, protocols and valuable insights from other clinicians. An absolutely essential tool for the practicing health professional.

123 pages   ISBN 0-929167-07-4 $44.95

Apple-A-Day Press
Dedicated to the Healing of the Whole Person

Important News! Our web site www.apple-a-daypress.com offers additional health-enhancing services including Lab Tests, Tried 'N True Nutritional Programs, and Natural Resources (health building products) to bring you more tools for optimal health.

ORDER FORM

BOOKS & TAPES

- The Weight Is Over* (hardback) (ISBN 0-929167-19-8) ....$27.95 _____ $_____
- The Weight Is Over* (paperback) (ISBN 0-929167-xx-x)................................$21.95 _____ $_____
- Passion Play* (ISBN 0-929167-20-1)..$21.95 _____ $_____
- The Pro-Vita! Plan for Optimal Nutrition* (ISBN 0-929167-05-8) ....$21.95 _____ $_____
- Conquer Candida -- Restore Your Immune System* (ISBN 0-929167-00-7)..........$15.95 _____ $_____
- Breast Health -- Women's Health Discourse ....$9.95 _____ $_____
- The Next Step to Greater Energy* (ISBN 9-929167-04-X)...............................$16.95 _____ $_____
- Your Liver -- Your Lifeline!* (ISBN 0-929167-06-6) ....$14.95 _____ $_____
- The Healing Triad (2 CD set)...$19.95 _____ $_____
- Cooking with Brooke ....$11.00 _____ $_____

FOR THE HEALTH PROFESSIONAL

- A Guidebook to Clinical Nutrition...$21.95 _____ $_____
- Systemic Nutrition/Herbology Training Program (cassettes & manual) ....$159.00 _____ $_____
- Blood Chemistry & Clinical Nutrition (ISBN 0-929167-07-4) ....$44.95 _____ $_____

SCLEROLOGY

- Insights in the Eyes: An Introduction to Sclerology* (ISBN 9-929167-11-2)................$19.95 _____ $_____
- The Art & Science of Sclerology Certification Course (list $699) ....$399.00 _____ $_____
- Sclerology Pens...$3.95 _____ $_____
- Sclerology Wall Chart* (Color) ....$19.95 _____ $_____
- Sclerology Wall Chart (Organs Depicted) ....$13.95 _____ $_____
- Sclerology Starter Package (book, video, chart) ....$49.00 _____ $_____
- Sclerology Interpretive CD-ROM ....$199.00 _____ $_____
- The Art & Science of Sclerology Manual CD-ROM...$99.95 _____ $_____

* **Discount available with purchase of any combination of 12 or more of titles denoted with an asterix. Contact our office for more information.**

ORDER SUBTOTAL $_____
TAX (if applicable) $_____
S&H, COD $_____
TOTAL $_____

Name _____ Date _____

Address _____

City/State/Zip _____

Phone _____ E-mail_____

Method of Payment ☐ Check ☐ Credit Card

Name on card_____

Card # _____

Exp. Date_____

Signature _____

Order on the Internet at: www.apple-a-daypress.com

Apple-A-Day Press 1500 Village West Drive, Suite 77 Austin, TX 78733	**E-mail:** apple-a-day@austin.rr.com	**Phone:** 512-328-3996 **Toll Free:** 877-442-7753 **Fax:** 512-263-7787